Addressing Systemic Racism and Disparate Mental Health Outcomes for Youth of Color

Editors

LISA R. FORTUNA
CHERYL S. AL-MATEEN
LISA M. CULLINS
W. DAVID LOHR

CHILD AND ADOLESCENT PSYCHIATRIC CLINICS OF NORTH AMERICA

www.childpsych.theclinics.com

Consulting Editor
JUSTINE LARSON

April 2022 • Volume 31 • Number 2

ELSEVIER

1600 John F. Kennedy Boulevard • Suite 1800 • Philadelphia, Pennsylvania, 19103-2899

http://www.theclinics.com

CHILD AND ADOLESCENT PSYCHIATRIC CLINICS OF NORTH AMERICA Volume 31, Number 2
April 2022 ISSN 1056–4993, ISBN-13: 978-0-323-98765-3

Editor: Megan Ashdown
Developmental Editor: Arlene Campos

Child and Adolescent Psychiatric Clinics of North America (ISSN 1056-4993) is published quarterly by Elsevier Inc., 360 Park Avenue South, New York, NY 10010-1710. Months of issue are January, April, July, and October. Business and Editorial Offices: 1600 John F. Kennedy Boulevard, Suite 1800, Philadelphia, PA 19103-2899. Periodicals postage paid at New York, NY and additional mailing offices. Subscription prices are $358.00 per year (US individuals), $869.00 per year (US institutions), $100.00 per year (US & Canadian students), $399.00 per year (Canadian individuals), $895.00 per year (Canadian institutions), $459.00 per year (international individuals), $895.00 per year (international institutions), and $200.00 per year (international students). International air speed delivery is included in all *Clinics* subscription prices. All prices are subject to change without notice. **POSTMASTER:** Send address changes to *Child and Adolescent Psychiatric Clinics of North America*, Elsevier Health Sciences Division, Subscription Customer Service, 3251 Riverport Lane, Maryland Heights, MO 63043. **Customer Service: 1-800-654-2452 (U.S. and Canada); 314-447-8871 (outside U.S. and Canada). Fax: 314-447-8029. E-mail:** JournalsCustomer Service-usa@elsevier.com **(for print support) or** journalsonlinesupport-usa@elsevier.com **(for online support).**

Reprints. For copies of 100 or more of articles in this publication, please contact the Commercial Reprints Department, Elsevier Inc., 360 Park Avenue South, New York, New York 10010-1710 Tel.: 212-633-3874; Fax: 212-633-3820, E-mail: reprints@elsevier.com.

Child and Adolescent Psychiatric Clinics of North America is covered in *MEDLINE/PubMed (Index Medicus), ISI, SSCI, Research Alert, Social Search, Current Contents,* and *EMBASE/Excerpta Medica.*

Contributors

CONSULTING EDITOR

JUSTINE LARSON, MD, MPH, DFAACAP
Medical Director, Schools and Residential Treatment, Consulting Editor, Child and Adolescent Psychiatric Clinics of North America, Sheppard Pratt , Rockville, Maryland

EDITORS

LISA R. FORTUNA, MD, MPH
Professor of Psychiatry, Department of Psychiatry and Behavioral Sciences, University of California, San Francisco, Zuckerberg San Francisco General Hospital and Trauma Center, San Francisco, California

CHERYL S. AL-MATEEN, MD
Professor of Psychiatry and Pediatrics, Virginia Commonwealth University School of Medicine, Richmond, Virginia

LISA M. CULLINS, MD
Attending Physician, Emotion and Development Branch, National Institute of Mental Health, National Institutes of Health, Bethesda, Maryland

W. DAVID LOHR, MD
Professor of Pediatrics, Division of Child and Adolescent Psychiatry and Pediatric Psychology, University of Louisville School of Medicine, Louisville, Kentucky

JOEL SLACK
President, Slack Consulting, LLC, Montgomery, Alabama

PAIGE GAINES
Sane Jane Inc, Atlanta, Georgia

AUTHORS

MARGARITA ALEGRÍA, PhD
Disparities Research Unit, Massachusetts General Hospital, Departments of Medicine and Psychiatry, Harvard Medical School, Boston, Massachusetts

YOHANIS LEONOR ANGLERO, MD
Instructor of Psychiatry, Harvard Medical School, Boston Children's Hospital, Boston, Massachusetts

LILANTHI BALASURIYA, MD
National Clinician Scholars Program, Yale University School of Medicine, New Haven, Connecticut

TAMI D. BENTON, MD
Psychiatrist-in-Chief, Department of Child and Adolescent Psychiatry and Behavioral Sciences, Children's Hospital of Philadelphia, Associate Professor of Psychiatry, Perelman School of Medicine, University of Pennsylvania, Philadelphia, Pennsylvania

HERNÁN CARVENTE-MARTINEZ, BS
Founder/CEO, Healing Ninjas, Inc., Queens, New York

JANG CHO, MD
Cultivate Psychiatry, Yakima, Washington

ANGÉLICA CLAYTON, BA
Program in the History of Medicine and Science, Yale University, New Haven, Connecticut

NIKEEA COPELAND-LINDER, PhD, MPH
Co-Director, Center for Diversity in Public Health Leadership Training, Kennedy Krieger Institute, Baltimore, Maryland; Assistant Professor, Department of Psychiatry and Behavioral Sciences, Johns Hopkins School of Medicine

KARISSA DIMARZIO, MS
Department of Psychology, Center for Children and Families, Florida International University, Miami, Florida

ELIZABETH DOHRMANN, MD
Child and Adolescent Psychiatrist, Los Angeles County Department of Mental Health, Juvenile Justice Mental Health Program, Los Angeles, California

LISA R. FORTUNA, MD, MPH
Professor of Psychiatry, Department of Psychiatry and Behavioral Sciences, University of California, San Francisco, Zuckerberg San Francisco General Hospital and Trauma Center, San Francisco, California

KIMBERLY GORDON-ACHEBE, MD
Department of Psychiatry, Division of Child and Adolescent Psychiatry, University of Maryland School of Medicine, Baltimore, Maryland

ALEXA HOOBERMAN
Tufts University School of Medicine Boston, Massachusetts

ROYA IJADI-MAGHSOODI, MD, MSHPM
Assistant Professor-in-Residence, Division of Population Behavioral Health, Semel Institute for Neuroscience and Human Behavior, University of California, Los Angeles, Department of Psychiatry and Biobehavioral Sciences, David Geffen School of Medicine, University of California, Los Angeles, Health Service Research and Development (HSR&D) Center for the Study of Healthcare Innovation, Implementation and Policy (CSHIIP), VA Greater Los Angeles Healthcare System, Los Angeles, California

KAMILAH JACKSON, MD, MPH
Medical Director, PerformCare, Robbinsville, New Jersey

SHERYL H. KATAOKA, MD, MSHS
Professor Emeritus, Division of Population Behavioral Health, Semel Institute for Neuroscience and Human Behavior, University of California, Los Angeles, Los Angeles, California

QORTNI LANG, MD
NYU Grossman School of Medicine, NYU Langone Health, NYC Health + Hospital - Bellevue Medical Center, NYU Child Study Center, New York, New York

RUPINDER K. LEGHA, MD, PC
President, Los Angeles, California

PAMELA A. MATSON, PhD, MPH
Department of Pediatrics, Johns Hopkins School of Medicine, Department of Population, Family, and Reproductive Health Sciences, Johns Hopkins Bloomberg School of Public Health, Baltimore, Maryland

COURTNEY MCMICKENS, MD, MPH, MHS
Associate State Medical Director, North Carolina, Eleanor Health, Greensboro, North Carolina

SHAVON MOORE, MD
Assistant Clinical Professor, Department of Psychiatry, University of California, San Diego, San Diego, California

SHANKAR NANDAKUMAR, MD
Baylor College of Medicine, Houston, Texas

VINH-SON NGUYEN, MD
Baylor College of Medicine, Houston, Texas

ISABEL SHAHEEN O'MALLEY, BA
Disparities Research Unit, Massachusetts General Hospital, Boston, Massachusetts

MICHELLE V. PORCHE, EdD
Associate Professor, Department of Psychiatry and Behavioral Sciences, Zuckerberg San Francisco General Hospital and Trauma Center, University of California, San Francisco, San Francisco, California

ALEJANDRA POSTLETHWAITE, MD
Assistant Clinical Professor, UCSD Health Sciences, Neighborhood Healthcare, California

ERIC RAFLA-YUAN, MD
Voluntary Assistant Clinical Professor, Department of Psychiatry, University of California, San Diego, San Diego, California

BARBARA ROBLES-RAMAMURTHY, MD
Assistant Professor, Department of Psychiatry and Behavioral Sciences, University of Texas Health San Antonio, San Antonio, Texas

EUGENIO M. ROTHE, MD
Professor of Psychiatry, Herbert Wertheim College of Medicine, Florida International University, FIU Health Miami, Miami, Florida; Herbert Wertheim College of Medicine/Florida International University, Coral Gables, Florida

ARTURO SANCHEZ-LACAY, MD
BronxCare/Columbia University, BronxCare Hospital Center, Bronx, New York

NEHA SHARMA, DO, DFAACAP
Assistant Professor, Department of Psychaitry, Tufts University School of Medicine, Tufts Medical Center, Boston, Massachusetts

AMALIA LONDOÑO TOBÓN, MD
Postdoctoral Research Fellow, National Institutes of Health, National Institute on Minority Health and Health Disparities, Bethesda, Maryland

MARINA TOLOU-SHAMS, PhD
Professor, Department of Psychiatry and Behavioral Sciences, Zuckerberg San Francisco General Hospital and Trauma Center, University of California, San Francisco, San Francisco, California

MARIA TRENT, MD, MPH
Bloomberg Professor of American Health and Pediatrics, Department of Pediatrics, Johns Hopkins School of Medicine, Department of Population, Family, and Reproductive Health Sciences, Johns Hopkins Bloomberg School of Public Health, Johns Hopkins University, Baltimore, Maryland

ANNIE SZE YAN LI, MD
NYU Grossman School of Medicine, NYU Langone Health, NYC Health + Hospital - Bellevue Medical Center, NYU Child Study Center, New York, New York

PHILLIP YANG, MA
Joe R. and Teresa Lozano Long School of Medicine, University of Texas Health San Antonio, San Antonio, Texas

ANDREA S. YOUNG, PhD
Department of Psychiatry and Behavioral Sciences, Division of Child and Adolescent Psychiatry, Johns Hopkins School of Medicine, Baltimore, Maryland; Department of Mental Health, Johns Hopkins Bloomberg School of Public Health

LINDSAY YUEN, BA
University of California, Irvine School of Medicine, Irvine, California

HASIYA E. YUSUF, MBBS, MPH
Post-doctoral Fellow, Department of Pediatrics, Johns Hopkins School of Medicine, Baltimore, Maryland

JENNY ZHEN-DUAN, PhD
Disparities Research Unit, Massachusetts General Hospital, Department of Medicine, Harvard Medical School, Boston, Massachusetts

Contents

> In this framework, we synthesize the results of studies addressing racial/ethnic disparities in children's mental health through 4 domains hypothesized to impact minoritized children and their families: (1) policies, (2) institutional systems, (3) neighborhoods/community system, and (4) individual/family-level factors. We focus on children and adolescents, presenting findings that may impact mental health outcomes for major racial/ethnic groups In North America: Black/African American, Latinx, Asian, and American Indian youth. We conclude by suggesting areas for needed research, including whether certain domains of influence demonstrate differential impact for inequities reduction depending on the youth's race/ethnicity.

> Data from the US Department of Education clearly documents the chronic and persistent disproportionality of negative educational outcomes for students of color. To move closer to an antiracist system that provides all youth with the resources, protections, and opportunities to which they are entitled through public education, we recommend that mental health clinicians understand the social determinants of education; become familiar with the historical legacy of inequity in schools; identify current trends of racial disparities in education; engage in opportunities for antiracist school transformation; and reflect on their personal practices in providing access, diagnosis, and treatment to underresourced and minoritized youth.

> Suicide rates continue to increase among children and adolescents in the United States, with suicide remaining the second leading cause of death for youth aged 10 to 24 years of age. Most studies of suicide among

Black, Indigenous, and other Youth of Color (BIPOC youth) experience racism from a young age. These experiences have both immediate and long-term impacts on their health and wellbeing. Systemic racism contributes to the inequitable distribution of health resources and other social determinants of health, creating barriers to accessing care. Substance use disorders and sexual/nonsexual risk behaviors have been linked to experiences of racism in BIPOC youth. The legacy of generational racial trauma can frame behaviors and attitudes in the present, undermining health and survival in this group. BIPOC youth also face difficulties navigating spheres characterized as white spaces. Ethnic-racial socialization may promote resilience and help with coping in the context of racial stress. While many professional health organizations have embraced dismantling racism, a shift in the narrative on racial values will be critical for preventing adversity and achieving health equity for BIPOC youth.

This paper unpacks the legacy of racism and white supremacy in American child psychiatry, connecting them to current racist inequities, to reimagine an antiracist future for the profession, and to serve all children's mental health body and soul. History reveals how child psychiatry has neglected and even perpetuated the intergenerational trauma suffered by minoritized children and families. By refusing to confront racial injustice, it has centered on white children's protection and deleted their role in white supremacist violence. An antiracist future for the profession demands a profound historical reckoning and comprehensive reimagining, a process that this paper begins to unfold.

Supporting the mental health of youth who identify as Black, Indigenous, or Persons of Color (BIPOC) continues to be a challenge for clinicians and policymakers alike. Children and adolescents are a vulnerable population, and for BIPOC youth, these vulnerabilities are magnified by the effects of structural, interpersonal, and internalized racism. Integration of psychiatric care into other medical settings has emerged as an evidence-based method to improve access to psychiatric care, but to bridge the gap experienced by BIPOC youth, care must extend beyond medical settings to other child-focused sectors, including local governments, education, child welfare, juvenile legal systems, and beyond. Intentional policy decisions are needed to incentivize and support these systems, which typically rely on coordination and collaboration between clinicians and other stake-holders. Clinicians must be trauma-informed and strive for structural competency to successfully navigate and advocate for collaborative systems that benefit BIPOC youth.

Children rely heavily on their parents for guidance and support throughout development. When parental support is hindered by racial discrimination, poverty, trauma, and acculturative family distancing, barriers to a child's success are cultivated. It is imperative that providers of children and families address racial and cultural concerns in a humble, curious manner. Cultural adaptations to family-based care can lead to stronger outcomes with families.

This article describes the history of race relations and the rapidly changing racial topography of the United States. The authors address the history of racism and discrimination experienced by minority populations and immigrants of color and the psychological effects on these populations and describe the risk factors and protective factors that come into play when individuals are faced with experiences of discrimination and racism. They describe the process of ethnic-racial identity development and the different styles of ethnic-racial socialization and cultural orientation. Ultimately, it explains the importance of ethnicity and race in the psychotherapeutic encounter.

CHILD AND ADOLESCENT PSYCHIATRIC CLINICS

SERIES OF RELATED INTEREST
Psychiatric Clinics of North America
https://www.psych.theclinics.com/
Pediatric Clinics of North America
https://www.pediatric.theclinics.com/

THE CLINICS ARE AVAILABLE ONLINE!
Access your subscription at:
www.theclinics.com

Preface

Cultivating Solutions for Disparities in Mental Health Services and Outcomes Among Minoritized Youth

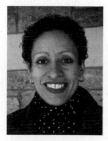 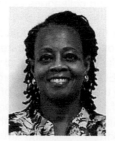 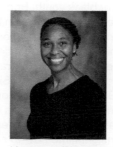 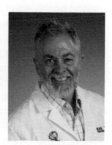

| Lisa R. Fortuna, MD, MPH | Cheryl S. Al-Mateen, MD | Lisa M. Cullins, MD | W. David Lohr, MD |

Editors

Despite national attention to the problem, disparities in mental health remain for minoritized youth of color in the United States. This special *Child and Adolescent Psychiatric Clinics of North America* issue is a comprehensive collection of articles, offering diverse perspectives for examining racialized disparities in child and adolescent mental health and inspiring solutions. This issue of the *Child and Adolescent Psychiatric Clinics of North America* offers insights from various disciplines, including education, pediatrics, and psychiatry and psychology, to highlight social, historical, and systemic issues important to recognize as foundational for cultivating tenable pathways to addressing disparities in clinical care. The authors share how child-serving systems of care can be improved to better serve youth of color, by focusing on the structural and social determinants of mental health inequities and by informing how our clinical care can be more responsive to the needs of youth and their experiences.

The first article by Alegria and colleagues grounds readers in a framework for "Understanding and addressing racial and ethnic disparities in children's mental health." The articles that follow focus on specific mental health and substance use care disparities faced by black and other minoritized youth, people of color, and within specific systems of care and health services. Kataoka and colleagues examine both racial disparities in the educational system and the opportunities to improve mental health services in schools. "Suicide among minoritized and marginalized youth" by Benton reviews the existing literature to help us begin to understand the alarming increase in suicide among youth of color. Fortuna and colleagues offer a review of health

Child Adolesc Psychiatric Clin N Am 31 (2022) xiii–xv
https://doi.org/10.1016/j.chc.2022.02.001
1056-4993/22/© 2022 Published by Elsevier Inc.

services research and insights into dismantling inequities in substance use services and outcomes for racially minoritized adolescents, including an intersectional identities perspective.

"Focusing on racial, historical, and intergenerational trauma and resilience," by Fortuna and colleagues, offers solutions for systems serving children and families who have experienced cumulative traumatic experiences. Li and colleagues discuss the need for cultural and structural humility in addressing disparities in our systems of care disparities in mental health services. "The impact of systemic racism on health and well-being of youth," by Trent and colleagues, reviews this important and timely literature for all of our youth. Legha and colleagues acknowledge the historical underpinnings of systemic racism and committing to an antiracist approach to achieve mental health equity for black youth. Robles and colleagues explore the opportunities and challenges inherent in both community mental health and collaborative care approaches. Sharma and colleagues explore the impact of culture, race, and racism on parenting, recognizing the importance of family-based care in this work. Rothe and Escobar examine immigration and racial identity in clinical practice. Finally, the issue includes an introduction by the RESPECT Institute of Georgia featuring the personal story of Paige Gaines to illustrate how the personal story of overcoming barriers is essential in the transformative process of healing and recovery.

By considering these major areas affecting minoritized youth mental health, this special issue offers insights into how to address social and structural inequities that perpetuate disparate clinical practice and outcomes for black and other minoritized children, youth, and their families. We have enjoyed bringing this compilation of articles to you and hope you also find this issue as compelling and necessary for effective clinical practice as we do.

Lisa R. Fortuna, MD, MPH
Department of Psychiatry and
Behavioral Sciences
University of California San Francisco
San Francisco, CA, USA

Zuckerberg San Francisco General Hospital
Department of Psychiatry 7M
1001 Potrero Avenue
San Francisco, CA, USA

Cheryl S. Al-Mateen, MD
Virginia Commonwealth University School of Medicine
PO Box 980489
Richmond, VA 23298, USA

Lisa M. Cullins, MD
Emotion and Development Branch
National Institute of Mental Health
9000 Rockville Pike, Building 10 4C438
National Institutes of Health
Bethesda, MD 20892, USA

W. David Lohr, MD
Division of Child & Adolescent Psychiatry & Pediatric Psychology
University of Louisville School of Medicine
200 E. Chestnut Street
Bingham Clinic, Louisville
KY 40202, USA

E-mail addresses:
lisa.fortuna@ucsf.edu (L.R. Fortuna)
cheryl.al-mateen@vcuhealth.org (C.S. Al-Mateen)
lisa.cullins@nih.gov (L.M. Cullins)
william.lohr@louisville.edu (W.D. Lohr)

A Personal Story

The RESPECT Institute of Georgia was created by mental health advocate, Joel Slack, who, after sharing his story of mental health challenges, treatment, and recovery to nearly 450,000 people worldwide, realized that standing up in front of people and utilizing lived experiences to educate others was therapeutic. His organization supports participants in developing the skills necessary to transform their experiences with mental health or substance use challenges and cross-disabilities into inspirational and educational presentations.

Following the training, the RESPECT Institute of Georgia Outreach Team facilitates speaking engagements for the graduates to share their stories statewide to diverse audiences. To date, the RESPECT Institute of Georgia graduates have shared their stories to more than 175,000 listeners in Georgia. Empowered by learning to share their stories, the RESPECT Institute of Georgia graduates report they feel more confident and in control of their life experiences. They give back to their community by sharing hope with fellow citizens who experience similar challenges.

The RESPECT Institute of Georgia is funded by the Georgia Department of Behavioral Health and Developmental Disabilities and works in partnership with the Georgia Mental Health Consumers Network and Slack Consulting. For more information about the RESPECT Institute of Georgia, please contact Joel Slack at joelslack@earthlink.net.

The following personal story by Ms Gaines was shared on October 25, 2021 for the 68th Annual Meeting of the American Academy of Child and Adolescent Psychiatry for the Systems of Care Committee's Special Program: Addressing Racially Disparate Outcomes in Child Serving Systems of Care: A Call for Child and Adolescent Psychiatry.

PAIGE GAINES: "MY STEPS TO RECOVERY"

Growing up, I had a beautiful family, amazing parents, and one brother. We lived in a beautiful brick home, which was always filled with excitement and joy. Besides all of my school and family activities, I spent Saturdays as a star soccer player, always elated in victory. These memories will forever be with me.

Another memory that will forever be with me is being only 10 years old, when I had my first panic attack. And I would have many more. As they continued traumatizing me, getting through middle school became difficult. Mean girls, silly boys, and the stress of school proved to be too much. At the age of 11, I began slipping into isolation and then depression. These dark days and nights felt endless, leaving me hopeless and frightened of my own mind.

I had the typical teenage drama, even an attitude, but I found myself arguing with my mom more often than not. Before I knew what was happening, my mom had sent me to live with my aunt. I recall sitting alone, with my feet dangling over the edge of a small bed, with two small windows behind me. As the sunlight peered through the blinds, I made a decision. A final decision. At the age of 12, I tried to end my life.

When I was returned to my home, it was no longer the happy place I had remembered. And quickly it turned into a nightmare after a relative came to visit and he

Child Adolesc Psychiatric Clin N Am 31 (2022) xvii–xx
https://doi.org/10.1016/j.chc.2022.01.006
1056-4993/22/© 2022 Published by Elsevier Inc.

molested me. This triggered my depressive symptoms and worsened my suicidal ideations. Six long years of this sexual abuse took a toll on my well-being, mentally, emotionally, spiritually, and physically.

Although I endured the unrelenting pain accompanied by depression, I smiled my way through prom, homecoming, and Friday night football games. But my teenage years were spent filled with silent tears and constant thoughts of death.

At 18, I was a college student, and I started living a careless drug and alcohol lifestyle. It was certainly not a party, like I thought. I began to self-medicate in order to cope with feelings of sadness and desperation. At 21, I was a college dropout consumed with debt and eviction notices. My mood swings and related outbursts were always followed by darkness, which were followed by psychosis.

One day, I found myself in a public psychiatric ward. The double doors of that psychiatric ward welcomed me with screaming patients, prickling needles, and a lot of staff gossip. As I shuffled through the dimly lit hall, a male guard awaited me for a strip down. A gown was tossed my way as I stood naked, trembling to cover myself. I spoke not a word as they pierced me with needles, leaving my arms bruised.

Another male nurse with an aura of joy grabbed my hand with such assurance that I will never forget his simple words, "You're special. The hard part is over. You are going to be more than fine." I never saw him again, but he gave me some sense of hope. It is truly amazing how kind words can take the edge off of some of the pain. Moments later, I was taken by ambulance to another hospital, but this one was a private hospital.

I remained silent and followed the instructions of the director. As we walked through the long halls, something became very clear to me. I was the only one who looked like me. This made me feel alone, and before any treatment even started, I was doubting if anyone would understand me. I was black, and they were not! And my doubts became a reality. No one seemed to understand that in my culture, the African American culture, emotional issues are strictly dealt with in secrecy, stern talk, and definitely with no acknowledgment of "mental illness." We are taught to fight any demons by trusting in the church and engaging God as a form of treatment. Considering that only a small percentage of credentialed mental health professionals are black, it's no wonder I felt out of place. I was never comfortable making casual conversation while my peers chatted as if we were on a lunch break. They were casual and comfortable talking about their psychiatric problems; I was embarrassed and needed to get right with God.

On my second day, I met with my psychiatrist. Once again, he was white, and I was black. He was a man, and I was a woman. I could not help but wonder how on earth he could relate to my secrets. In my culture, we don't share our secrets with "outsiders." And what if my family found out about my secrets because I had told a white psychiatrist rather than my black minister. And how was a psychiatrist going to help me when my understanding of getting better, since childhood, was hinged on dropping to my knees and praying? I was skeptical: therapy or medications, it all seemed foreign to me. I had learned that sad thoughts were those of the devil.

I must say that this psychiatrist worked hard to overcome the cultural barriers. Would it have been more comfortable for me to have had a black psychiatrist? I think yes. But when it is not possible, white mental health professionals should learn the skills to navigate the color barriers. To make a long story short, we discussed my secrets, and I began to find relief. I finally had answers as to why my life had been turned upside down. I now knew the language to communicate with family and friends on how to best help me. We discussed symptoms: intense mood swings, heavy alcohol and drug abuse, suicidal ideation, anxiety, and depression. I was then given a diagnosis of bipolar disorder. I define this diagnosis as one day you are enjoying jumping on the bed and having a good time, elated and free, and then days or weeks later you find yourself hiding under your bed scared, sad, hopeless, and exhausted. This had been my life.

At the age of 23, after finding some understanding and becoming stabilized, I still found myself unstable, in toxic relationships, and hypersexual. Although in treatment, my symptoms remained, and while still struggling, one day it all caught up with me.

On my 25th birthday, while depressed, I made a decision that would change my life forever. As the night progressed and the drinking increased, I found myself one mile from home when I drove my car into a large drainage ditch filled with boulders. As I sat in my car, I asked myself many questions, one being, "How on earth did I get here?"

Arrested for a DUI, I spent my 25th birthday in jail sleeping on a steel bench. The following morning, when I woke up, I was ready for change. I made a decision to seek recovery. I no longer wanted to be intoxicated. I no longer wanted to live in darkness.

I began with baby steps. Daily 5-minute meditation sessions. Daily 10-minute reading sessions. Twenty minutes of writing. I continued to exercise my brain and began seeing the benefits of taking my mental health seriously. These small changes made all the difference. In addition to my own efforts, my family was on board, and therapy guided us through these difficult times. We used coping skills and correct language to communicate symptoms and steps to recovery. My steps to recovery.

As I grew, my recovery became a reality, and I was living a life some people said I might never have. I rebuilt my support system around people who looked like me. You must understand, I needed doctors who were culturally competent. I needed them to grasp the challenge of educating not just me, but my family as well. And my family was black, too!

In the following months, I again was transferred to a new psychiatrist. Unbeknownst to me, he was black. I will never forget our conversation and the intense approach he took while educating me on the process of medication. I was at once skeptical for obvious reasons, one being a conversation I had with my mom. She agreed on me getting help while in the same breath saying, "Do not let them put you on any medication, WE do not do that." We, in this case, is the black community. Remember when I said I was told to pray? I was always being told to turn my worries and struggles over to the Lord.

As the years passed, and with my newly built support system in my corner, I was guided through the many stages of recovery. One year from the beginning of my recovery, I had overcome obstacles I once considered impossible.

I purchased my first car, moved into my own place, became a certified peer specialist, and held a 9 to 5 job. I even received a phone call from the University of Arkansas asking me to tell my story of recovery to a group of teens living with mental health challenges. WOW, look at what recovery can do!

Today, I am a peer specialist, a college graduate, and a business owner. I am the founder and CEO of 911 Sane Jane (https://www.911sanejane.com/), an organization geared toward providing the black and brown community with resources and a place to share their own story. I continue my work in the community as an advocate. Through transparency, I have been able to educate and support those who look like me and share similar challenges. In addition to advocacy, I provide mental health education to teachers, law enforcement, social workers, and others in the community.

As I think about my past accomplishments, my list of goals continues to grow. I wish to develop a curriculum for peers and parents to assist them in the recovery process. I would also like to travel the world to share hope and recovery with those in need.

To my peers, I say, KEEP GOING! Recovery is possible and rewarding. Go for your dreams! If you can dream it, you can do it!

To the mental health professionals, I say, thank you for inviting me to share my story with you. Listening to stories of recovery will give you more insight into what it takes to build a relationship with us. Whether we are black or white, our goal should always be to listen to each other and learn from each other.

Thank you for listening to my story.

Joel Slack, President
Slack Consulting, LLC
7931 Long Acre Street
Montgomery, AL 36116, USA

Paige Gaines
911Sane Jane Inc
245 North Highland Avenue Northeast
Suite 230 #908
Atlanta, GA 30307, USA

E-mail addresses:
joelslack@earthlink.net (J. Slack)
sj@911sanejane.com (P. Gaines)

Framework for Understanding and Addressing Racial and Ethnic Disparities in Children's Mental Health

Margarita Alegría, PhD[a,b,c,]*, Isabel Shaheen O'Malley, BA[a],
Karissa DiMarzio, MS[d], Jenny Zhen-Duan, PhD[a,b]

KEYWORDS

- Racial and ethnic disparities • Youth mental health • Equity

KEY POINTS

- *Policies:* We present the evidence of programs proposed within the Pursuing Equity in Mental Health Act (H.R. 1475) and related policies that would expand services and mitigate racial and ethnic disparities among youth.
- *Systems:* Systemic sources of disparities are pervasive and complex, with the impact of separate institutions often compounding the negative effects of others; this necessitates both multi-level and multi-system interventions to effectively improve the mental health trajectories for youth of color.
- *Neighborhoods:* Interventions directed at the physical and social environment whereby youth of color reside can advance opportunities for prevention and remediation in mental health problems and mitigate racial and ethnic disparities.
- *Individual:* Childhood adversities can alter bodies at a molecular level and change the way the body's stress response system works. Growing research has elucidated potential biological pathways linking stress and adversity and mental health outcomes among youth of color.

BACKGROUND

The 2020 United States Census[1] indicates population growth among minoritized children. The child population is currently 25.7% Latinx, 13.9% Black or African American,

[a] Disparities Research Unit, Massachusetts General Hospital, 50 Staniford St, Suite 830, Boston, MA 02114, USA; [b] Department of Medicine, Harvard Medical School, 25 Shattuck St, Boston, MA 02115, USA; [c] Department of Psychiatry, Harvard Medical School, 401 Park Drive, 2 West, Room 305, Boston, MA 02215, USA; [d] Department of Psychology, Center for Children and Families, Florida International University, 11200 SW 8th St, AHC-1, Miami, FL 33199, USA
* Corresponding author. Massachusetts General Hospital Disparities Research Unit, Department of Medicine, 50 Staniford Street, Suite 830, Boston, MA 02114.
E-mail address: malegria@mgh.harvard.edu

Child Adolesc Psychiatric Clin N Am 31 (2022) 179–191
https://doi.org/10.1016/j.chc.2021.11.001
1056-4993/22/© 2021 Elsevier Inc. All rights reserved.

childpsych.theclinics.com

5.5% Asian, 1.4% American Indian and Alaska Native, 15.1% "two or more races", and 10.9% "some other race alone."[1] Rising trends in diversity are especially important for clinicians given the significant racial/ethnic disparities documented in mental health disorders prevalance[2] and access to needed services.[3,4] For example, Latinx children use in-school mental health services at a significantly lower rate than their white counterparts.[5] Similarly, significant differences by race/ethnicity were detected in out-of-school service use for each diagnostic group, illustrating unrelenting disparities in care.

The fact that disparities have persisted across settings emphasizes the importance of identifying and understanding mechanisms and alternatives to traditional care. In this article, we elucidate the importance of a multi-pronged coordinated approach to restructuring mental health prevention and services for youth of color to tackle these inequities and ensure all children have optimal mental and emotional development. We draw on theoretic models[6,7] of the underlying mechanisms, with some evidence of what seems to amplify or reduce these disparities. The integrative risk and resilience model[8] builds on Garcia-Coll's seminal framework[9] to describe ways racial/ethnic minorities' mental health outcomes are shaped by factors at different ecological levels. Bernard and colleagues add those adversity-specific frameworks to understand child mental health outcomes need to capture racism, historical oppression, traumas, and social conditions (eg, poverty) that racial/ethnic minority youth confront.[10]

An important first step to achieving equity across domains is recognizing that racism is a fundamental cause of inequities.[11,12] Dr. Camara-Jones posits that "racism is a system of structuring opportunity and assigning value based on the social interpretation of how one looks (which is what we call 'race'), that unfairly disadvantages some individuals and communities, unfairly advantages other individuals and communities, and saps the strength of the whole society through the waste of human resources."[13] We also follow Camara-Jones' conceptualization of health equity, as "the assurance of the conditions for optimal health for all people."[14] The American Academy of Pediatrics acknowledged the fundamental role of racism in inequities[15] and the importance of pediatric health professionals' ability to engage in preventive strategies to optimize the way we design and conduct clinical care, workforce development, professional education, systems engagement, and research, to reduce the health effects of structural, personally mediated, and internalized racism.[15] This is an important paradigm shift—from blaming children and families of color, to now focusing attention to the policies and systems that create and perpetuate inequities in mental health services and outcomes.

The Framework. As illustrated in **Fig. 1**, racial/ethnic disparities in children's mental health can be understood within 4 domains: 1) policies, laws, and regulations; 2) institutional systems; 3) neighborhoods/community system; and 4) individual and family-level factors. This model follows work we and others have published emphasizing how these 4 domains and life course perspective call for the study of human lives within the context of time, age, and social patterns that affect individual trajectories (see **Fig. 1**).[16] One key principle is that of "linked lives," which assumes that individuals are interdependent with families and peers and are impacted by what happens in their communities and how the institutional systems and policy can influence their well-being. Applied to the problem of racial/ethnic discrimination-related stressors and health inequities by Gee and colleagues,[17] the concept of linked lives implies that when one person encounters discrimination in housing or employment access, it can have ripple effects across their close social network, and over generations, that can impact family, peers, and even neighborhood experiences in mental health. To illustrate the framework, we begin with a discussion of the 4 domains and how each

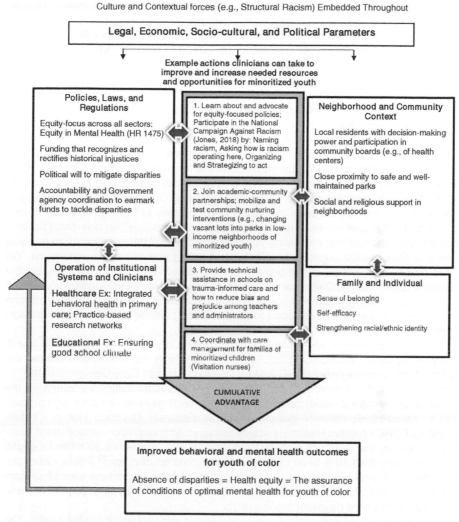

Fig. 1. Sociocultural framework for understanding and addressing racial and ethnic disparities in children's mental health.

compounds experiences of disadvantage among minority populations. We then transition to a greater focus on modifiable factors that can promote change across domains.

Policies, Laws, and Regulations

A review of mental health and mental health care disparities research (across the lifespan)[18] identified a need for studies focusing on policy-level predictors of mental health care disparities. Contemporary health disparities result from "the cumulative impact of centuries of systemic exclusion from legal protections, and restricted access to opportunities and resources that are protective of health" (p. 308).[6] Understandably, more than 5 years are needed for most macro interventions to witness a reduction in disparities.[6] For example, ParentCorps and Earned Income Tax Credit seemed to have no change in the short term (adolescence) but demonstrated a significant change in mental health and reducing disparities in the longer term (adulthood). A policy is not likely to reduce racial/ethnic mental health disparities without explicitly prioritizing resources and opportunities for racial/ethnic groups[19] who have been underserved and systematically underresourced due to structural racism. Prior work has described public policies' impact on improving the mental health of youth of color and reducing racial/ethnic disparities.[20,21] Persistent issues in the enactment of equity-focused policies include the lack of earmarked funding, technical assistance, and lack of political imperative.

Modifiable Factors for Policy Change. In an overview of recent policies that explicitly address racism in children's mental health services, Alvarez and colleagues[22] concluded that the policy with the most potential for broad and lasting impact is the Pursuing Equity in Mental Health Act (H.R. 1475) which was passed in the House (5/12/2021) and is awaiting a vote in the Senate as of October 2021 (Congress.gov, HR 1475). The primary purpose of this act is to respond to the mental health needs of youth of color. Stakeholders have discouraged "standalone" (ie, one-time) policies to address racial equity in improving youth mental health[23] because they can relegate new practices to silos outside of mainstream funding and delivery mechanisms. Yet these limited-term policies have been important demonstrations for establishing the evidence base, such as California's Mental Health Services Act (Proposition 63) which was associated with increased access to care for Latinx and Asian youth and reduced disparities,[24] and serves as the basis for implementing further reform to improve treatment quality.

Develop infrastructure for youth-centered models of integrated behavioral health and primary care. The Pursuing Equity in Mental Health Act would also amend the Public Health Service Act (42 USC 290dd) Integrated Health Care Demonstration Program by adding $100 million in grants for interprofessional health care teams for the provision of behavioral health care in primary care settings in areas with a high proportion of racial/ethnic minority groups, such as Federally Qualified Health Centers (FQHCs). FQHCs receive Health Research Services Administration federal grant funding to improve the health of underserved populations and serve 30 million people, including more than 10% of all children, mostly children of color.[25] Policy directions for reducing mental health disparities through integrated care include allocating state Medicaid funding for Accountable Care Organizations,[26] bundled payments, and other integrated care payment mechanisms.[19]

Increase funding for research on racial and ethnic minority youth mental health. The largest funding authorization in the Pursuing Equity in Mental Health Act is $650 million annually for 5 years to the National Institute of Minority Health and Health Disparities (NIMHD). The act authorizes additional funds for the NIH ($100 million annually for 5 years) to build relations with communities and conduct clinical research on racial or ethnic disparities in physical and mental health. Both are sorely needed given the shortage of evidence-based psychosocial interventions for minority youth.[23,27] This policy is likely to improve mental health given that a large portion of culturally appropriate evidence-based interventions was developed or adapted with funding from the NIMHD. This act also requires the NIH Director to partner with the National Academies of Medicine to conduct a study on research gaps in racial/ethnic mental health disparities, including structural racism.

Expand health insurance coverage and eligibility requirements. The Children's Health Insurance Program (CHIP) and Medicaid through the Affordable Care Act improved coverage, access, and quality of care, and narrowed disparities between White children and Hispanic and Black children across all 3 categories.[28] The Early

Screening Detection and Treatment (EPSDT) benefit under Medicaid enables Medicaid-eligible children to have access to preventive, diagnostic, and treatment services for physical, mental, and dental conditions. Insurance coverage, combined with improving patient education and availability of community clinics, has reduced service disparities across racial/ethnic groups, including removing the disparity between Latinx and non-Latinx whites, while African Americans were still 10% less likely to receive care compared with non-Latinx whites with the same insurance.[29] Expanding Medicaid eligibility in states that have opted out of ACA Medicaid expansion[19] might help reduce inequities, given the large numbers of uninsured Latinx families living in such states.[30]

Operation of the Institutional Systems

Systemic sources of disparities are pervasive and complex, with the impact of separate institutions often compounding the negative effects of the others. For example, educational attainment has been shown to be an important contributing factor to one's health[31]; however, youth of color face several barriers to learning (eg, harsher discipline) that diminish the quality of their educational experience and that are associated with negative educational outcomes.[32] This can result in long-term mental health consequences that are more likely to go unmet for these youth due to additional systemic barriers in the health care system.[15] Moreover, it perpetuates a cyclical pattern of adversity and inequality that compounds poor mental health functioning of youth over time. This is important given that mental health concerns beginning in childhood and adolescence can cause problems that persist into adulthood and increase health care expenditures and economic burden.[33]

Educational systems. Schools play a decisive role in youth mental health outcomes, with those that offer caring and nurturing relationships[34] and school safety[35] demonstrating better outcomes than those missing these characteristics. But students' perception of their school environment has been shown to vary by race/ethnicity, with Black youth more likely to report negative experiences than their White counterparts attending these same schools.[36] Importantly, experiences of discrimination and racism, even indirectly as a bystander, can be deleterious to the health of students of color[15,32] and represent yet another threat to these students' educational experiences. One source of these negative experiences is the differential treatment in school disciplinary action, which may account for almost half of the Black/White student gap in suspensions and expulsions.[37]

Juvenile justice and child welfare systems. Degrees of disadvantage differ according to the stage (ie, arrest vs probation) and group of youth being observed, but the consensus is that the juvenile justice system is less favorable to racial/ethnic minority youth compared to whites.[38] More evidence exists to suggest this is especially true for Black and Latinx youth, while significantly less work has focused on the impact on American Indian/Native Alaskan, Asian, and Native Hawaiian/Pacific Islander youth. In addition to the juvenile justice system, racial/ethnic minorities are also disproportionately referred to child protective services, particularly Black families. Dettlaf & Boyd[39] highlight the importance of the intersectionality between race and socioeconomic status (SES), noting the associated risk factors (eg, increased financial and parenting stress) that increase families' vulnerability to maltreatment and child welfare contact. The juvenile justice system presents with an inordinate number of challenges that racial/ethnic minority youth and their families face in everyday life, which, when compounded by experiences of institutional racism and structural barriers that prevent these youth and families from obtaining equitable support, create the perfect storm for perpetuating systems of oppression.

Modifiable system factors. Effectively addressing systemic disparities would require a multi-level approach and, to eliminate disparities in mental health, the reformation of multiple systems. While this represents a considerable undertaking, the literature has presented promising avenues for advancement. For example, efforts to reduce racial/ethnic disparities in the child welfare system have emphasized the importance of establishing long-term community collaborations, promoting workforce diversity, and enhancing cultural competency.[40,41] Data-driven decision-making was also noted as an essential component due to needed adjustments as systems changed over time.[40]

Role of Neighborhoods and Communities

The vital role of neighborhood residence has been tied to mental health outcomes. Both the physical environment (eg, pollution) and the social environment (eg, exposure to violence) can change neurodevelopment, modifying epigenetic variation and biological systems that interact with development.[42] For that reason, environmental variables operating at the expansive societal level and more proximal neighborhood level have been labeled "the exposome".

Economic hardship. A plethora of studies links neighborhood socioeconomic conditions and safety with children's mental health outcomes.[43] For example, Coulton and colleagues[44] report how rises in vacant housing, neighborhood unemployment rates, and extreme racial segregation seem related to upsurges in child maltreatment rates. Similarly, Hurd and colleagues[45] found that greater neighborhood poverty and unemployment rates predicted greater internalizing symptoms due to lower social support and cohesion.

Discrimination. Discrimination experienced in the neighborhood has shown a deleterious and pervasive effect on the mental health of minoritized youth.[46–48] But again, there is evidence that suggests that the discrimination experienced by minoritized youth might vary by racial/ethnic groups,[49] with visible minority status and receiving context dynamically impacting youth mental health outcomes. Everett and colleagues[50] found higher reports of perceived discrimination among Black youth, lower rates among Asian youth, and similar rates for Latinx youth as contrasted to non-Latinx White youth. In their study, discrimination had significant effects on depressive symptoms but not on anxiety symptoms. Work by others[46,51] has found statistically significant relationships of discrimination on anxiety disorders in Latinx youth. Of interest is the finding that discrimination might have a more corrosive effect on majority than minority groups, partly explained by lacking mechanisms to cope with discrimination.

Exposure to violence. Neighborhood violence also seems to have negative consequences for children's cognitive performance and self-regulatory behavior.[52,53] Neighborhood violence seems to modify the social interactions in disadvantaged communities, with increased experiences of discrimination that augment neighborhood inequities in mental health outcomes.[46] Evidence also shows that moving out of violent environments alters developmental consequences, with children who departed from extremely violent neighborhoods (to less violent ones) demonstrating improvements in cognitive skills and mental health.[54] More recent research using social network analysis has found[55] that patterns of everyday urban mobility are better predictors of homicides than fixed neighborhood disadvantage, with suggested explanations by authors including drug activity, gun crime prevalence, and interpersonal friction.

Social capital and collective efficacy. The physical and social conditions of a child's neighborhood impact the mental health of the child's caregivers, the parental interactions with children, and mental health outcomes of White and Black children.[56] Whether the effects of neighborhood social capital and collective efficacy are seen when Latinx children are older remains unknown. Also of significance is the interaction of maternal depression and neighborhood social capital for behavior problems in adolescents. For example, Delany-Brumsey and colleagues[57] showed that living in neighborhoods with higher levels of social capital diminished the association between maternal depression and adolescent behavior problems. Latinx children's neighborhood sense of community has also been identified as a buffer for children's behavior outcomes.[58]

Ethnic density. Who resides in the neighborhood matters. After adjustments for the material deprivation of the neighborhood, Latinx immigrant ethnic density was found[59] to predict Latinx immigrant youth's lower odds of depression onset. However, this protective effect was not found for non-immigrant Latinx youth. The potential of Latinx immigrants to be a psychosocial resource in the neighborhood seems to offset the stress Latinx immigrants face, possibly explaining positive mental health outcomes. In parallel, greater concentrations of Black residents and stable residents in Black neighborhoods have been associated with fewer internalizing symptoms among Black adolescents, potentially explained by youth's perceptions of greater social support and cohesion.[45]

Modifiable neighborhood factors. There has been a meteoric growth in the literature identifying modifiable neighborhood factors linked to well-being and mental health outcomes. We draw attention to the physical and social environment, as it conveys opportunities for prevention and remediation in mental health and mitigation of racial and ethnic disparities in youth mental health outcomes. Being able to identify how crime decline has impacted disparities in children's mental health outcomes is also sorely needed. Work by van de Weijer and colleagues[60] evaluated 2 large-scale data resources to identify environmental factors associated with well-being. In longitudinal analyses, the researchers[60] found that housing stock, neighborhood income, core neighborhood characteristics, livability, and socioeconomic conditions of the neighborhood in childhood were all associated with well-being in adulthood. This is important as residential segregation by income is increasing in the United States.[61] Once researchers adjusted for individual and neighborhood income, only neighborhood safety and greater percentage of land dedicated to greenhouse horticulture were found to be significantly related to well-being.

Individual and Family Factors

Biological impact of stress and adversity. Researchers have more recently focused on ways that stress "gets under the skin,"[62] altering biology leading to mental health outcomes and disparities. Most of the current risk and resilience research has focused on ways stressors affect the hypothalamic–pituitary–adrenal (HPA) axis and how these are linked to mental health outcomes. Studies have found flatter awakening cortisol slopes among Latinx and African American youth, compared to their White peers.[63,64] Flatter awakening slopes, or cortisol not appropriately peaking during awakening, is indicative of HPA dysregulation and has been previously linked to poor health outcomes and early death.[65] Similar patterns of HPA dysregulation have been observed among American Indian young adults, perhaps indicative of heightened rates of chronic adversities during childhood.[66] Experiencing discrimination has also been linked with HPA axis hyperactivity among racially diverse youth[67] and young adults.[68]

Emotion regulation. Aspects of emotion regulation, such as effortful control, can protect Latinx youth exposed to stressors from poor mental health outcomes.[69] Latinx immigrant youth, who may experience acculturation- and assimilation- related stressors, are more likely to have high levels of emotion regulation if they have positive social relationships, have a sense of purpose, and are adaptable to environmental demands.[70] One prospective study found that Black youth with good emotion regulation skills showed adaptive cortisol levels irrespective of the degree of psychosocial stressors experienced.[71]

Modifiable individual and family factors. A protective factor particularly salient to youth of color is having a strong sense of their own racial and/or ethnic identity.[51,72,73] Positive perceptions of one's race/ethnicity have been linked to improved self-esteem, better academic outcomes, and decreased internalizing and externalizing problems.[51,72] For example, in their cross-sectional investigation, Zhen-Duan and colleagues[73] found that Puerto Rican girls who had greater acceptance of their ethnic identity reported higher self-concept despite experiencing elevated levels of cultural stress. Social networks within and outside of the family unit have been shown to facilitate racial/ethnic identity promotion[74] via socialization messages.[72] An important commonality underlying these constructs is that they are all central to how youth perceive and experience the world around them. Unfortunately, achieving acceptance of one's racial/ethnic identity can be challenging when messages of positivity being conveyed by close friends and family are directly opposed by surrounding messages in the external environment.

SUMMARY

Mental health disparities among children and youth continue to widen,[2] highlighting the need to engage in efforts alternative to traditional care. Clinicians hold critical roles in evoking change at the policy, institutional, neighborhood, and individual levels that we have outlined in this article. Future work will require centering attention on policies to address structural racism and work toward equity.[75] Clinicians can use their expertise to advocate for equity-focused policies and further the development of methods to assess ways structural racism impacts youths' mental health.[76] Clinicians can also initiate, or be part of, community and clinical interventions to develop "nurturing neighborhoods"[77] (eg, to minimize physical and social toxic exposure, strengthen prosocial and resiliency outcomes, and ensure psychological safety and well-being for minoritized children) in an effort to promote healthy development. Clinicians can provide consultations for community-based prevention and intervention work that would help mitigate racial/ethnic disparities. Specific to mental health delivery, the field should be moving toward integrated/collaborative care models, with youth-centered models at the forefront, which have been found to reduce disparities by making care more accessible to marginalized communities.[25]

CLINICS CARE POINTS

Pitfalls - DON'T...
1. Fail to conceptualize childrens' mental health needs within the context of policies and laws that perpetuate the cycles of oppression and marginalization.
2. Approach clinical care without addressing the intersecting systemic risks that maintain the cyclical pattern of adversity.
3. Ignore neighborhood and community characteristics that contribute to clinical presentations and oppress families and youth of color.
4. Overlook ways stressors can be embodied and carried throughout the development of children of color.

Pearls – DO...

---

1. Advocate for policies and practices that are more responsive to addressing racism and mental health issues afflicting youth of color.
2. Support an overhaul of institutions that youth of color come into contact with to address biases and practice a nurturing neighborhood and community to ensure mental health development.
3. Use your voice to support more modifiable neighborhood and systemic factors that will promote mental health.
4. Encourage youth of color to tap into cultural factors that will buffer stressors both biologically and psychologically.

DISCLOSURE

We would like to acknowledge the National Institute on Minority Health and Health Disparities (Grant number: 1R01MD014737-01A1) and the National Institute of Mental Health (Grant number: R01MH117247).

REFERENCES

1. US Census Bureau. Percentage distribution of race and hispanic origin by age group: 2010 and 2020. Available at: https://www.census.gov/content/dam/Census/library/stories/2021/08/improved-race-ethnicity-measures-reveal-united-states-population-much-more-multiracial-figure-5.jpg.
2. Ghandour RM, Sherman LJ, Vladutiu CJ, et al. Prevalence and treatment of depression, anxiety, and conduct problems in US children. J Pediatr 2019;206:256–67.e3.
3. Barksdale CL, Azur M, Leaf PJ. Differences in mental health service sector utilization among african American and caucasian youth entering systems of care programs. J Behav Health Serv Res 2010;37(3):363–73.
4. Cummings JR, Druss BG. Racial/ethnic differences in mental health service use among adolescents with major depression. J Am Acad Child Adolesc Psychiatry 2011;50(2):160–70.
5. Locke J, Kang-Yi CD, Pellecchia M, et al. Ethnic disparities in school-based behavioral health service use for children with psychiatric disorders. J Sch Health 2017;87(1):47–54.
6. Brown AF, Ma GX, Miranda J, et al. Structural interventions to reduce and eliminate health disparities. Am J Public Health 2019;109(S1):S72–8.
7. Alvidrez J, Castille D, Laude-Sharp M, et al. The National Institute on minority health and health disparities research framework. Am J Public Health 2019;109(S1):S16–20.
8. Suárez-Orozco C, Motti-Stefanidi F, Marks A, et al. An integrative risk and resilience model for understanding the adaptation of immigrant-origin children and youth. Am Psychol 2018;73(6):781–96.
9. García Coll C, Lamberty G, Jenkins R, et al. An integrative model for the study of developmental competencies in minority children. Child Dev 1996;67(5):1891–914.
10. Bernard DL, Calhoun CD, Banks DE, et al. Making the "C-ACE" for a culturally-Informed Adverse childhood experiences framework to understand the pervasive mental health impact of racism on Black youth. Journ Child Adol Trauma 2020. https://doi.org/10.1007/s40653-020-00319-9.
11. Bailey ZD, Feldman JM, Bassett MT. How structural racism works — Racist policies as a Root cause of U.S. Racial health inequities. N Engl J Med 2021;384(8):768–73.

12. Clark R, Anderson NB, Clark VR, et al. Racism as a stressor for African Americans. A biopsychosocial model. Am Psychol 1999;54(10):805–16.
13. Jones CP. Toward the Science and practice of Anti-racism: Launching a National Campaign against racism. Ethn Dis 2018;28(Suppl 1):231–4.
14. Jones CP. Systems of power, axes of inequity: parallels, intersections, braiding the strands. Med Care 2014;52(10 Suppl 3):S71–5.
15. Trent M, Dooley DG, Dougé J. The impact of racism on child and adolescent health. Pediatrics 2019;144(2):e20191765.
16. Alegria M, Alvarez K, Pescosolido BA, Canino G. A socio-cultural framework for mental health and substance abuse service disparities. In: Sadock B, Sadock V, Ruiz P, editors. Kaplan and Sadock's Comprehensive Textbook of Psychiatry2, 10th edition. Philadelphia: Wolters Kluwer; 2017. p. 4377–887.
17. Gee GC, Walsemann KM, Brondolo E. A life course perspective on how racism may be related to health inequities. Am J Public Health 2012;102(5):967–74.
18. Cook BL, Hou SS, Lee-Tauler SY, et al. A review of mental health and mental health care disparities research: 2011-2014. Med Care Res Rev 2019;76(6): 683–710.
19. Cook B, Zuvekas S, Chen J, et al. Assessing the individual, neighborhood, and policy predictors of disparities in mental health care. Med Care Res Rev 2017; 74(4):404–30.
20. Perrin JM, Duncan G, Diaz A, et al. Principles and policies to strengthen child and adolescent health and well-being. Health Aff (Millwood) 2020;39(10):1677–83.
21. National Academies of Sciences. In: Bonnie RJ, Backes EP, editors. Engineering, and Medicine. *The Promise of adolescence: Realizing Opportunity for all youth.* The National Academies Press; 2019. https://doi.org/10.17226/25388.
22. Alvarez K., Cervantes P.E., Nelson K.L., Seag D.E., Horwitz S. and Hoagwood K.E., Structural racism and the children's mental health service system: Recommendations for policy and practice change, J Am Acad Child Adolesc Psychiatry, *In-press.*
23. Harris TB, Udoetuk SC, Webb S, et al. Achieving mental health equity: children and adolescents. Psychiatr Clin North Am 2020;43(3):471–85.
24. Ashwood JS, Kataoka SH, Eberhart NK, et al. Evaluation of the mental health services act in Los Angeles county. Rand Health Q 2018;8(1):2.
25. Health resources and services Administration. Health center program: impact and growth. Bureau of primary health care. 2021. Available at: https://bphc.hrsa.gov/about/healthcenterprogram/index.html. Accessed October 14, 2021.
26. National Association for State Health Policy. National Academy for state health policy. Resources for states to address health equity and disparities. 2019. Available at: https://nashp.org/resources-for-statesto- address-health-equity-and-disparities/#toggle-id-2.
27. Pina AA, Polo AJ, Huey SJ. Evidence-based psychosocial interventions for ethnic minority youth: the 10-year update. J Clin Child Adolesc Psychol 2019;48(2): 179–202.
28. Hayes SL, Riley PR, Radley DC, et al. Fewer uninsured children, less disparity, and Keeping it that way. Commonw Fund. Available at: https://www.commonwealthfund.org/blog/2017/fewer-uninsured-children-less-disparity-and-keeping-it-way. Accessed October 14, 2021.
29. Alegria M, Lin J, Chen C-N, et al. The impact of insurance coverage in diminishing racial and ethnic disparities in behavioral health services. Health Serv Res 2012;47(3 Pt 2):1322–44.

30. Bailey A, Hayes K, Katch H, et al. Medicaid is key to building a system of comprehensive substance use care for low-income people. Center on Budget and Policy Priorities 2021;1–20. https://www.cbpp.org/research/health/medicaid-is-key-to-building-a-system-of-comprehensive-substance-use-care-for-low. [Accessed 14 October 2021].

31. Hamad R, Elser H, Tran DC, et al. How and why studies disagree about the effects of education on health: a systematic review and meta-analysis of studies of compulsory schooling laws. Soc Sci Med 2018;212:168–78.

32. Benner AD, Wang Y, Shen Y, et al. Racial/ethnic discrimination and well-being during adolescence: a meta-analytic review. Am Psychol 2018;73(7):855–83.

33. Copeland WE, Wolke D, Shanahan L, et al. Adult functional outcomes of common childhood psychiatric problems: a prospective, longitudinal study. JAMA Psychiatry 2015;72(9):892–9.

34. Wang M-T. School climate support for behavioral and psychological adjustment: testing the mediating effect of social competence. Sch Psychol Q 2009;24(4):240–51.

35. Konishi C, Miyazaki Y, Hymel S, et al. Investigating associations between school climate and bullying in secondary schools: multilevel contextual effects modeling. Sch Psychol Int 2017;38(3):240–63.

36. Bottiani JH, Bradshaw CP, Mendelson T. Inequality in Black and white high school students' perceptions of school support: an Examination of race in context. J Youth Adolesc 2016;45(6):1176–91.

37. Owens J, McLanahan SS. Unpacking the drivers of racial disparities in school suspension and expulsion. Social Forces 2020;98(4):1548–77.

38. Spinney E, Cohen M, Feyerherm W, et al. Disproportionate minority contact in the U.S. juvenile justice system: a review of the DMC literature, 2001–2014, Part I. J Crime Justice 2018;41(5):573–95.

39. Dettlaff AJ, Boyd R. Racial disproportionality and disparities in the child welfare system: why Do they exist, and what can Be Done to address them? ANNALS Am Acad Polit Social Sci 2020;692(1):253–74.

40. Duarte CS, Summers A. A three-pronged approach to addressing racial disproportionality and disparities in child welfare: the Santa Clara County example of leadership, collaboration and data-driven decisions. Child Adolesc Social Work J 2013;30(1):1–19.

41. Pryce J, Lee W, Crowe E, et al. A case study in public child welfare: County-level practices that address racial disparity in foster care placement. J Public child welfare 2019;13(1):35–59.

42. National Academies of Sciences, Engineering, and Medicine. Division of behavioral and social Sciences and education; board on children, youth, and families; Committee on Fostering healthy mental, emotional, and behavioral development among children and youth. Fostering healthy mental, emotional, and behavioral development in children and youth: a National Agenda. National Academies press (US). 2019. Available at: http://www.ncbi.nlm.nih.gov/books/NBK551842/. Accessed October 14, 2021.

43. Ludwig J, Duncan GJ, Gennetian LA, et al. Neighborhood effects on the long-term well-being of low-income adults. Science 2012;337(6101):1505–10.

44. Coulton CJ, Richter FG-C, Korbin J, et al. Understanding trends in neighborhood child maltreatment rates: a three-wave panel study 1990-2010. Child Abuse Negl 2018;84:170–81.

45. Hurd NM, Stoddard SA, Zimmerman MA. Neighborhoods, social support, and african american adolescents' mental health outcomes: a multilevel path analysis. Child Dev 2013;84(3):858–74.
46. Alegria M, Shrout PE, Canino G, et al. The effect of minority status and social context on the development of depression and anxiety: a longitudinal study of Puerto Rican descent youth. World Psychiatry 2019;18(3):298–307.
47. Marcelo AK, Yates TM. Young children's ethnic-racial identity moderates the impact of early discrimination experiences on child behavior problems. Cultur Divers Ethnic Minor Psychol 2019;25(2):253–65.
48. Pascoe EA, Richman LS. Perceived discrimination and health: a meta-analytic review. Psychol Bull 2009;135(4):531–54.
49. Bourque F, van der Ven E, Malla A. A meta-analysis of the risk for psychotic disorders among first- and second-generation immigrants. Psychol Med 2011;41(5):897–910.
50. Everett BG, Onge JS, Mollborn S. Effects of minority status and perceived discrimination on mental health. Popul Res Policy Rev 2016;35(4):445–69.
51. Delgado MY, Nair RL, Updegraff KA, et al. Discrimination, Parent-adolescent conflict, and peer Intimacy: Examining risk and resilience in Mexican-origin youths' adjustment trajectories. Child Dev 2019;90(3):894–910.
52. Sharkey P. The acute effect of local homicides on children's cognitive performance. Proc Natl Acad Sci U S A 2010;107(26):11733–8.
53. Sharkey PT, Tirado-Strayer N, Papachristos AV, et al. The effect of local violence on children's attention and Impulse control. Am J Public Health 2012;102(12):2287–93.
54. Sharkey P, Sampson RJ. 13. Violence, cognition, and neighborhood inequality in America. In: Social Neuroscience: Brain, Mind, and society. Harvard University Press; 2015. p. 320–39.
55. Levy BL, Phillips NE, Sampson RJ. Triple disadvantage: neighborhood networks of everyday urban mobility and violence in U.S. Cities. Am Soc Rev 2020;85(6):925–56.
56. Pachter LM, Auinger P, Palmer R, et al. Do parenting and the Home environment, maternal depression, neighborhood, and chronic poverty affect child behavioral problems differently in different racial-ethnic groups? Pediatrics 2006;117(4):1329–38.
57. Delany-Brumsey A, Mays VM, Cochran SD. Does neighborhood social capital buffer the effects of maternal depression on adolescent behavior problems? Am J Community Psychol 2014;53(0):275–85.
58. Lardier DT, MacDonnell M, Barrios VR, et al. The moderating effect of neighborhood sense of community on predictors of substance use among Hispanic urban youth. J Ethn Subst Abuse 2018;17(4):434–59.
59. Lee M-J, Liechty JM. Longitudinal associations between immigrant ethnic density, neighborhood Processes, and Latino immigrant youth depression. J Immigr Minor Health 2015;17(4):983–91.
60. van de Weijer MP, Baselmans BML, Hottenga J-J, et al. Expanding the environmental scope: an environment-wide association study for mental well-being. J Expo Sci Environ Epidemiol 2021;1–10. https://doi.org/10.1038/s41370-021-00346-0.
61. Reardon SF, Bischoff K. Income inequality and income segregation. Am J Sociol 2011;116(4):1092–153.
62. Blair C, Raver CC. Poverty, stress, and Brain development: new directions for prevention and intervention. Acad Pediatr 2016;16(3 Suppl):S30–6.

63. DEER LK, SHIELDS GS, IVORY SL, et al. Racial/ethnic disparities in cortisol diurnal patterns and affect in adolescence. Dev Psychopathol 2018;30(5): 1977–93.

64. DeSantis AS, Adam EK, Doane LD, et al. Racial/ethnic differences in cortisol diurnal Rhythms in a community Sample of adolescents. J Adolesc Health 2007;41(1):3–13.

65. Saxbe DE. A field (researcher's) guide to cortisol: tracking HPA axis functioning in everyday life. Health Psychol Rev 2008;2(2):163–90.

66. Johnson-Kwochka A, Bond GR, Becker DR, et al. Prevalence and quality of individual placement and support (IPS) supported employment in the United States. Adm Policy Ment Health 2017;44(3):311–9.

67. Huynh VW, Guan S-SA, Almeida DM, et al. Everyday discrimination and diurnal cortisol during adolescence. Horm Behav 2016;80:76–81.

68. Yip T, Smith P, Tynes M, et al. Discrimination and hair cortisol concentration among asian, latinx and white young adults. Compr Psychoneuroendocrinology 2021;6:100047. https://doi.org/10.1016/j.cpnec.2021.100047.

69. Taylor ZE, Jones BL, Anaya LY, et al. Effortful control as a mediator between contextual stressors and adjustment in Midwestern Latino youth. J Latina/o Psychol 2018;6(3):248–57.

70. Archuleta AJ. Newcomers: the contribution of social and psychological well-being on emotion regulation among first-generation acculturating Latino youth in the Southern United States. Child Adolesc Soc Work J 2015;32(3):201–90.

71. Kliewer W, Roid Quiñones K, Shields BJ, et al. Multiple risks, emotion regulation skill, and cortisol in low-income african American youth: a Prospective study. J Black Psychol 2009;35(1):24–43.

72. Jones SC, Neblett EW. Racial–ethnic protective factors and mechanisms in psychosocial prevention and intervention programs for Black youth. Clin child Fam Psychol Rev 2016;19(2):134–61.

73. Zhen-Duan J, Jacquez F, Sáez-Santiago E. Boricua de pura cepa: ethnic Identity, cultural stress and self-concept in Puerto Rican youth. Cult Divers Ethnic Minor Psychol 2018;24(4):588.

74. Williams JL, Tolan PH, Durkee MI, et al. Integrating racial and ethnic identity research into developmental understanding of adolescents. Child Development Perspect 2012;6(3):304–11.

75. Schor EL. Developing a structure of essential services for a child and adolescent mental health system. Milbank Q 2021;99(1):62–90.

76. Groos M, Wallace M, Hardeman R, et al. Measuring inequity: a systematic review of methods used to quantify structural racism. J Health Disparities Res Pract 2018;11(2). Available at: https://digitalscholarship.unlv.edu/jhdrp/vol11/iss2/13.

77. Biglan A, Hinds E. Evolving prosocial and sustainable neighborhoods and communities. Annu Rev Clin Psychol 2009;5(1):169–96.

Racial Disparities in the Education System

Opportunities for Justice in Schools

Elizabeth Dohrmann, MD[a,*], Michelle V. Porche, EdD[b],
Roya Ijadi-Maghsoodi, MD, MSHPM[c,d,e],
Sheryl H. Kataoka, MD, MSHS[f]

KEYWORDS

- Racial/ethnic disparities • School-based mental health • School segregation
- School discipline • School resource officers • Trauma-informed • Public education

KEY POINTS

- Racial disparities in the US education system are influenced by a long history of structural racism, not group differences between youth.
- Increasing community partnerships and reducing teacher bias, clinician bias, and exclusionary discipline are prime targets for system transformation.
- Mental health clinicians can support racial equity in schools by advocating for a trauma-informed developmental framework and self-reflecting on diagnostic treatment patterns.

INTRODUCTION

Most of the youth with mental health concerns in the United States obtain care through the US public school system.[1] Despite the importance of addressing the mental health needs of students from ethnic and racially diverse backgrounds, significant racial disparities persist in the US public school system, affecting academic outcomes, earning potential, and mental health disorder burden.[2–4] Although these disparities are endemic to the system, the challenges brought by COVID-19 have exacerbated the

[a] Los Angeles County - Department of Mental Health, Los Angeles, CA, USA; [b] Department of Psychiatry and Behavioral Sciences, University of California, San Francisco, 1001 Potrero Avenue, 7M16, San Francisco, CA 94110, USA; [c] Division of Population Behavioral Health, Semel Institute for Neuroscience and Human Behavior, University of California, Los Angeles, 760 Westwood Plaza, #A8-224, Los Angeles, CA 90095, USA; [d] Department of Psychiatry and Biobehavioral Sciences, David Geffen School of Medicine, University of California, Los Angeles, Los Angeles, CA, USA; [e] Health Service Research & Development (HSR&D) Center for the Study of Healthcare Innovation, Implementation & Policy (CSHIIP), VA Greater Los Angeles Healthcare System, Los Angeles, CA, USA; [f] Division of Population Behavioral Health, Semel Institute for Neuroscience and Human Behavior, University of California, Los Angeles, 760 Westwood Plaza, #48-240B, Los Angeles, CA 90024, USA
* Corresponding author. 16350 Filbert Street, Sylmar, CA 91342.
E-mail address: edohrmann@dmh.lacounty.gov

Child Adolesc Psychiatric Clin N Am 31 (2022) 193–209
https://doi.org/10.1016/j.chc.2022.01.001
1056-4993/22/© 2022 Elsevier Inc. All rights reserved.

burden faced by students of color. These students faced greater structural inequities and higher rates of traumatic stress at the start of the pandemic, followed by disproportionately higher barriers to instruction, high projected learning loss, and increased psychosocial burdens when compared with their White peers as the pandemic proceeded.[4–6] Communities of color also experienced a disproportionately higher rate of hospitalization and death due to COVID-19 and greater housing instability and unemployment, which can be negatively reflected in students' performance.[7–10]

In recognition of these additional burdens faced by youth of color and the essential role of education in case conceptualization, we suggest that mental health clinicians consider the social and structural factors influencing educational outcomes as *social determinants of education* (SDoE), expanding on Krieger's framework of social determinants of health.[11] We propose that SDoE include the child's neighborhood; the economic resources of the family and community; access to food, clothing, shelter, and health care; and exposure to sources of trauma, such as community or family violence, racism, police brutality, immigration trauma, sudden death, neglect, or abuse.[12,13] These factors contribute to persistent racial disparities in education. Addressing these disparities to move toward educational equity requires clinicians, educators, and school administrators to collaborate in reducing barriers and increasing supports for minoritized students through innovative policy and practice change.

The pursuit of school equity is grounded in the legal right of every child to enroll in the public school system and receive an accessible education in the least restrictive environment.[14] Teaching is structured to meet academic benchmarks, facilitate skill progression, and engage students in the learning process as demonstrated through outcomes such as academic achievement, graduation rates, attendance, and rates of discipline.[15] When youth are not able to access equitable educational opportunities, they are not equally valued or prepared for their role in civic life.

To equitably provide education for all students and ensure that minoritized youth living in underresourced communities can access the curriculum, public schools are legally required to support students and their families by linking them to services such as physical and mental health care, housing, and food assistance.[16,17] Schools in underresourced communities bear the brunt of a higher level of services needed with fewer community and school district resources. This disparity is largely due to a long history of redlining and redistricting, concentrating people of color in areas with lower property values, and perpetuating a cycle of reduced resources but greater need.[18] Such exclusion efforts in communities and voting districts have resulted in multigenerational disenfranchisement in housing, education, employment, and wealth building that have shaped the social determinants predicting academic and social outcomes.[18]

All of these determinants are linked to worsened educational outcomes in terms of academic performance and graduation rates. More than 1.3 million students who are unhoused—and disproportionately identified as LGBTQ+, Black, and Native American—often have multiple periods of school dropout.[19] Youth with at least one risk factor including minoritized racial or language status, household poverty, or single-parent home, are 66% more likely to drop out than students without one of these risk factors.[20] School dropout is also mediated by childhood psychiatric diagnoses, particularly conduct disorder and substance use, which are more commonly diagnosed in youth of color and may serve as proxies for more complex trauma-driven behaviors.[21,22]

Currently, most public school students are children of color, with greater than 51% identifying as minoritized students, with particular growth seen in Latinx, Asian, and multiracial student populations.[23] Minoritized students face the greatest barriers to educational equity and mental health care.[24] This is a clear call to action. What can mental health clinicians working within the school system do?

As clinicians, we can support our education colleagues in moving toward educational equity by highlighting the role of psychological well-being in promoting academic success and developing strategies to buffer the risks that arise from experiences of racial trauma.[3,15,25] In this article we review an abbreviated historical legacy of school inequity; identify current trends of racial disparities in education; discuss opportunities for antiracist school transformation; and implore clinicians to reflect on ways they can personally improve diagnosis and treatment of underresourced and minoritized youth.

THE HISTORICAL LEGACY OF A SEPARATE AND UNEQUAL EDUCATION SYSTEM

Slavery is fundamentally intertwined with the inception of the United States, and enslaved people were prohibited by law from any educational opportunities, including learning to read or write.[26] Following the Civil War, the Thirteenth and Fourteenth Amendments to the U.S. Constitution illegalized slavery and legislated that Black Americans held status as citizens with equal legal protections, respectively. However, in reaction to the brief period of Reconstruction, states rushed to create Jim Crow laws that siphoned away what little educational, occupational, and social opportunity Black Americans had. The US Supreme Court upheld a "separate-but-equal" paradigm in their Plessy vs Ferguson decision in 1090 that permitted the continued segregation of public spaces.[27] Decentralized school systems created separate and grossly underfunded facilities for Black Americans and other youth of color.

In 1909, the group later known as the National Association for the Advancement of Colored People (NAACP) issued a platform identifying the desegregation of American public schools as a primary legal focus.[28] NAACP attorneys brought multiple cases to trial, paving the way for the 1954 Brown vs Board of Education Supreme Court decision, which held that separate education was fundamentally unequal.[29] Segregation was no longer de jure in schools; however, it remained de facto throughout the country and particularly in the South, which doubled down on Jim Crow exclusion, violence, and intimidation of Black youth and families attempting to seek an integrated education.[30] Further complicating the integration process was the effective shutting out of Black teachers—who had provided rigorous instruction and socioemotional support to Black children in the face of legal opposition—from the White teaching workforce.[31] To this day there remains a missing "added value" of the benefits of same race teachers for Black and Latinx students.[32]

The pressure needed to enforce desegregation came from the Federal Civil Rights Act of 1964, which prohibited discrimination in federally funded programs and allowed for withholding of federal funds from noncompliant districts.[30] The same year the Department of Education Office for Civil Rights was created to engage in data collection and review. In 1965, the Elementary and Secondary Education Act (ESEA) was passed with the aim of providing federal funds to school districts serving impoverished students, to offset funding deficits from property tax revenue.[33] Mandated busing further advanced integration, although simultaneously and through the present, additional court decisions limiting desegregation efforts have dampened states' ability to further this process.[34]

As the primary federal law authorizing spending on K-12 schools, the ESEA was reauthorized most recently in December 2015 when it was renamed from "No Child Left Behind" (NCLB) to the "Every Student Succeeds Act" (ESSA). Despite intentions,

NCLB parameters resulted in penalizing schools serving underresourced students by focusing primarily on grade level testing, leading some schools to "teach to the test," lower standards, apply for waivers, or receive fewer federal dollars, compounding the funding problem for underresourced districts.[35] ESSA gives states more oversight and flexibility in terms of goals, consequences, and choice of outcome measurements; however, it also relies on individual states to determine how they will address equity without federal regulation.[36]

In recent decades school discipline policies have contributed to the "pushing out" of primarily minoritized students from schools, echoing earlier segregation. The use of zero-tolerance policies with automatic suspensions and expulsions originated during the 1980s in response to the "War on Drugs" and intensified following high-profile but rare events of school shootings.[37] Over time, these policies expanded in scope to include minor infractions such as dress code violations or subjective "defiance" from a student, leading to further widening of achievement gaps and increased promotion of mass incarceration of students of color.

School surveillance increased hand-in-hand with zero tolerance. Schools installed metal detectors, camera surveillance, and an increased police presence including School Resource Officers (SROs), leading some youth and educators to compare their school environment with jail.[38] Increased law enforcement presence is associated with worsened educational outcomes and increased carceral contact for minoritized students and those with disabilities.[39,40] Such funneling of youth out of schools through campus expulsions or arrests to the juvenile detention system has become known as the "school-to-prison pipeline" and remains a significant problem.[39,41]

RACIAL DISPARITIES IN US PUBLIC SCHOOLS

Although not an exhaustive list, several examples of racial disparities in schools that directly affect mental health outcomes include (1) use of a deficit model for school achievement; (2) higher rates of exclusionary discipline among children of color; and (3) disproportionate rates of adverse childhood experiences (ACEs) and disruptive behavior psychiatric diagnoses among children of color. As clinicians consider a patient's school history, awareness of these disparities can be critical in their assessment and ultimately how they intervene (see later section, A Path to Justice in the Education System).

Bias in the Classroom

The deficit model in education refers to the practice of attributing a student's academic or behavioral difficulties to a deficit within the student, their family, or their culture and often leads to reduced expectations.[42,43] Research demonstrates that educators engage in deficit thinking more often when working with students of color, students with disabilities, youth with lower socioeconomic backgrounds, or English learners, which paves the way for misinterpretation of behaviors or skills, overrepresentation in special education, and disproportionate use of exclusionary practices such as suspension and expulsion.[42–45]

Overrepresentation of minoritized and low-income students in special education has been described since the late 1960s.[46] Compellingly, recent data suggest that racial bias is the primary predictor: Black and Latinx youth are more often assigned to "lower status" disabilities such as Emotional Disturbance or Intellectual Disability that result in separate class settings than White youth, who are more likely to receive "higher status" disability categories that involve increased accommodations and services within the general education classroom.[46,47] In addition, these assignments increase as a function of the percentage of White youth in a school—for example, there is more exclusionary classroom push-out of minoritized youth when more White youth are enrolled.[46]

Implicit bias also has profound effects in the classroom. Higher aggregate rates of negative bias toward Black students compared with White peers from teachers is associated with higher suspension rates for Black students when compared with White students.[48] In addition, a longitudinal study of Latinx adolescents found that overt racial-ethnic discrimination is associated with rule-breaking behaviors (eg, cutting classes, lying, cheating) that were mediated by posttraumatic symptoms.[49] In addition, data suggest that school staff microaggressions insinuating that female, Black, or Latinx students are less capable than White male students are a powerful factor in driving students of color away from certain fields of study.[50]

Disparities in Exclusionary Discipline

Exclusionary practices such as suspensions and expulsions developed alongside mandated integration, targeting the removal of Black students.[37] Such disparate out-of-school discipline practices begin early: data from preschools show higher rates of suspensions and expulsions for Black preschoolers, especially Black boys, compared with their White counterparts, which continues today despite extensive awareness of this issue.[51] In fact, according to the 2017-2018 Civil Rights Data Collection, Black preschool children were suspended 2.5 times greater than their proportion in the preschool population. Similarly, American Indian/Alaskan Native and Multiracial preschool children were suspended 1.5 times greater than their proportions in the preschool population[52] (**Fig. 1**). These disproportionalities by race and ethnicity persist in K-12 schools, despite past studies that fail to demonstrate any differences in behavior between Black and White students.[53]

With heightened concerns about school safety and the increased presence of SROs, minor school disruptions and mental health incidents are increasingly managed by law enforcement. A recent scoping review found a lack of empirical evidence or

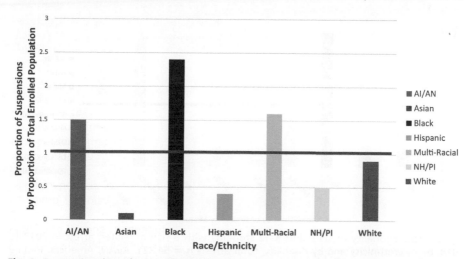

Fig. 1. Proportionality of US public preschool students with at least one out-of-school suspension in 2017 to 2018, by race/ethnicity, n = 2833. AI/AN, American Indian/Alaskan native; NH/PI, native Hawailan/Pacific Islander. (*Data from* the Office for Civil Rights, U.S. Department of Education, Civil Rights Data Collection. https://ocrdata.ed.gov/estimations/2017-2018. Accessed September 15, 2021.)

rigorous research evaluating the impacts of SROs in school mental health response.[54] On the other hand, studies indicate that the presence of SROs is associated with higher rates of exclusionary discipline and more referrals of youth of color and with disabilities to law enforcement.[39,55] These referrals and arrests are not evenly distributed and have increased in the past several years.[52] Across US K-12 public schools, American Indian/Alaskan Native, Black, and Native Hawaiian/Pacific Islander students are disproportionately represented in school-related arrests[52] (**Fig. 2**). In addition, youth with disabilities—many including youth of color—are disproportionately arrested.[52]

Adverse Childhood Experiences, Behaviors, and Mental Health Diagnosis

Viewing these racial disparities through a mental health lens, we conceptualize these chronic harms of daily discrimination in the classroom as forms of ACEs. ACEs are potent social determinants found to have both immediate and long-lasting effects on physical and mental health.[56] Minoritized youth have higher rates of exposure to ACEs than White peers, and youth detained in juvenile settings—who are disproportionally youth of color—have disturbingly high rates.[57,58] School-based racial microaggressions can exacerbate the impact of ACEs for Black youth and diminish psychological resources for resilience.[25]

Reactive behaviors associated with trauma exposure can be categorized by mental health professionals as disruptive behavior disorders (DBDs) such as oppositional defiant disorder and conduct disorder.[59,60] DBDs are stigmatized diagnoses that are applied frequently to Black and other youth of color, often at the expense of considering other diagnoses, such as posttraumatic stress disorder, attention-deficit/hyperactivity disorder (ADHD), or depressive or anxiety disorders, which are more commonly diagnosed and treated in White children.[21,61,62] Trauma and loss can play a large role not only in behavior but also in school attendance and academic outcomes among minoritized youth.[63,64] In acknowledging these potential effects, mental health clinicians can advocate for patients with a trauma history, thereby

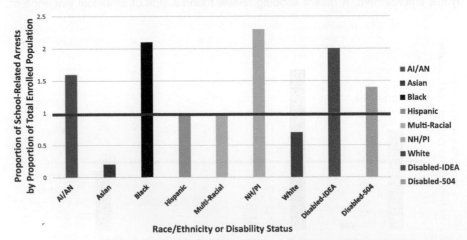

Fig. 2. Proportionality of US public K-12 students with a school-related arrest in 2017 to 2018, by race/ethnicity and by disability, total arrests n = 54,321. AI/AN, American Indian/Alaskan native; Disabled 504, students served under section 504 of the Rehabilitation Act of 1973; Disabled-IDEA, students served under the individuals with Disabilities Education Act; NH/PI, native Hawailan/Pacific Islander. (*Data from* the Office for Civil Rights, U.S. Department of Education, Civil Rights Data Collection. https://ocrdata.ed.gov/estimations/2017-2018. Accessed September 15, 2021.)

helping to build supportive school structures and an educational plan that takes into account the role of trauma on school behaviors and academic performance.

When behavioral manifestations of trauma are accurately diagnosed, the doors can open to more evidence-based treatments and deeper partnerships with caregivers.[21] Because of multiple factors, including the history of racism in mental health diagnostic labels, the process of psychiatric diagnosis for children who are referred for classroom behaviors or academic difficulties requires particular context sensitivity and family collaboration. For example, families of minoritized children in treatment of ADHD have described specific stages of engagement—from processing stigma to becoming advocates for their child to gaining empowerment through support and information— that are opportunities for clinicians to join families in this process more collaboratively.[65]

A PATH TO JUSTICE IN THE EDUCATION SYSTEM

Given our Nation's chronic and entrenched racial disparities in schools, we propose that a multilevel socioecological justice approach that extends beyond allocation of resources is essential to implementing an antiracist education system (**Fig. 3**).[66] This path to justice requires policy and structural changes, community voices at the table, and a whole school approach that recognizes the role of trauma and builds on the strengths and resilience of all students. Although we apply this framework to a limited discussion of social-emotional learning and disciplinary practices, similar ecological approaches can be applied to other areas of disparities in the education system such as school segregation and the use of high-stakes testing.[67] We take the position that this broad framework is essential to the work of mental health clinicians and actionable by us at all levels, albeit at a broader scope than clinicians often envision their role.

Policies to Foster Educational Justice

Policies at the local, state, and federal levels are needed to provide additional funding to underresourced schools serving minoritized students. Federal policies such as ESSA can potentially be used to reimagine education and their accountability systems. Instead of focusing on standardized test scores, which can be inherently biased, states can measure school climate and discipline practices by race and promote culturally responsive practices in their classrooms.

Congressional action can also invigorate local policy change. In 2018, Congress reevaluated the role of SROs on K-12 campuses and issued a report recommending

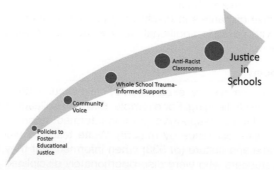

Fig. 3. Path to justice in the education system.

that schools reevaluate their safety plans to determine the necessity of SROs and hire those with backgrounds in child development, among other recommendations.[68] Since this report, several cities across the country have been reassessing their use of SROs and looking toward alternatives.

A recent example of this involves a series of resolutions by Los Angeles Unified School District. In 2007 the school board approved the Discipline Foundation Policy with the goal to reduce exclusionary discipline practices, later implementing a School Climate Bill of Rights in 2013 that went further to eliminate suspensions based on "willful defiance," implement Restorative Justice programming, develop a Positive Behavior Intervention and Support taskforce, and devise guidelines for SROs.[69] In 2021, largely in response to student activists and community members, the school board reallocated funding from the Los Angeles School Police Department to the Black Student Achievement Plan, which was developed in 2019 and expanded to support the hiring of school climate coaches, nurses, and counselors in schools serving predominantly Black students.[70]

Transforming Schools Through Community Voices

A promising approach with the potential to "disrupt inequality" in traditional educational systems is the *Community-Schools Model*, which calls for shared educational decision-making between district and school administrators and local communities.[71] The 4 pillars of this model—integration of mental health and social services with academics, family engagement, extended learning programs, and shared decision-making between school and community partners—have been shown to enhance positive youth development and school outcomes.

Whole-School Trauma-Informed Supports

Educational systems can benefit from comprehensive whole-school tiered approaches to health promotion, preventive services, and access to needed treatment, such as described in the Multi-Tiered Systems of Supports (MTSS) model.[72] We reframe the MTSS model for addressing racial disparities within a trauma-informed framework and invert the traditional triangle diagram to emphasize the importance of prevention (**Fig. 4**). Fallon and colleagues provide a comprehensive discussion of MTSS in promoting racial equity.[72]

As an example of a Tier 1 universal approach and alternative to exclusionary discipline, Restorative Justice (RJ) refers to a range of practices based on an acknowledgment of the impact of harm caused by a behavior on the harmed and the harmer; reconciliation between the two; and reintegration of the harmer into the community.[73] To date, the implementation process of RJ across school districts and states can vary widely, yielding mixed research findings.[74] Preliminary evidence, however, suggests that RJ can improve disparities in disciplinary practices, rates of misbehavior, and school climate, with possible additional positive effects on reducing bullying and school absenteeism.[75]

Antiracist Classrooms

The integration of racism history, exploration of child circumstances, and practitioner self-reflection can be challenging. For example, Blitz and colleagues found that implementation of a culturally responsive trauma-informed approach for elementary schools was met with resistance by majority White teachers who felt attacked as "insensitive" to race and culture (p. 533) when informed that they took a colorblind approach to the students who were disproportionately disciplined and doing poorly academically.[76] Yet impactful instruction of young children of color who have

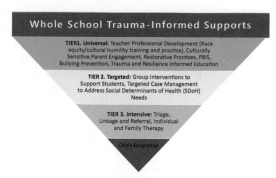

Fig. 4. Multi-tiered system of support (MTSS), adapted with a trauma-informed racial justice approach for schools. (*Adapted from* Lavelle C. and Kataoka S.H. Trauma Screening and Support: A Framework for Providing Comprehensive, Data Driven School Mental Health Services, *National Center for School Mental Health Annual Meeting*. Las Vegas, NV: October 2018, Presentation.)

experienced trauma depends on authentic relationships, trust building, and practice of cultural humility, which includes recognizing one's own identity and its impact in working with students and their families.[77] For this reason, it is important to account for racial trauma in designing antiracist and trauma-sensitive classrooms. Joseph and colleagues provide recommendations to educators for using critical race theory and ACEs frameworks to select nonpunitive responses to child behaviors.[78]

DEVELOPMENTAL CONSIDERATIONS ON THE PATH TO JUSTICE

Mental health professionals can offer significant contributions as advocates for developmentally informed school practices that may help bend the arc to more equitable outcomes. In addition to promoting these frameworks, we encourage clinicians to reflect on some particular challenges and opportunities embedded in each developmental stage as detailed in **Table 1**.

DISCUSSION

We have summarized some of the many educational disparities related to behavior and social-emotional well-being for students from preschool through high school, following a review of the history that has led us to this point. A persistent and disturbing trend in educational racial disparities is the practice of excluding youth of color, whether through exclusionary disability designation, exclusionary discipline, or bias in the classroom that can result in disengagement from school. As mental health clinicians in partnership with school and community stakeholders, we can play important roles in all levels of advocacy, research, and clinical care on a path toward educational justice.

Acknowledging the structural core of racial disparities in education and beyond, we can advocate for *policy changes* that directly address root causes of persistent inequities in these systems. Areas of focus include increasing funding for underresourced schools serving Black students; funding universal high-quality preschools for all children; mandating trauma-informed and antiracist practices for all school staff; limiting SROs on K-12 campuses as part of a commitment to reduced practice of exclusionary discipline; and funding ample after-school and year-round programming to provide structured, safe opportunities for continued growth and mastery, on both academic and socioemotional levels.

Table 1
Developmental considerations on the path to justice in the education system

School Level	Developmental Focus	Disparities	Path to Justice
Early Childhood Education (ECE)	• School readiness • Family involvement • Early social skills • SEL	• Lower quality ECE in low-income settings[79,80] • High rates of ECE suspension/expulsion of Black boys[51]	• Policies for universal preschool • Extend high-quality preschools for low-income and children of color, which can yield higher HS graduation rates, employment, home ownership[81] • Support teachers through the IECMHC model, teaming ECE staff with MH clinicians[82]
Elementary	• Academic skills • Social skills • Community building • Self-esteem	• Underresourced families have more barriers to school engagement, including work inflexibility, transportation, outside support, or immigration concerns[83] • Overrepresentation of White teachers in underresourced schools with challenges connecting to minoritized students[84]	• Positive reinforcement of strengths improves academic behaviors and reduces violent, sexual, substance use behaviors[85] • Parental engagement is associated with academic achievement[86] • School-based parental networks can improve engagement rates[84]
Secondary	• Individual and peer group identity building • Choosing educational/career path	• Bullying based on race disproportionately occurs in youth of color[87,88] • Black and Latinx youth are sorted into lower-achieving academic tracks[89]	• Evidence-based bullying prevention can decrease bullying in minoritized youth[90]

Abbreviations: SEL, social-emotional learning; HS, high school; IECMHC, infant and early childhood mental health consultation model.

A critical change in the *research framework* of school disparities involves the measurement of rates of racial discrimination and trauma in the school setting to better understand both risk factors and influences on subsequent emotional distress and academic failure.[91,92] Essential to the future of research in this and other areas is the development of research partnerships with school communities, using measures and practices that are meaningful to them. Increased emphasis should be placed on interventions and practices that have promising face validity in communities of color.

Clinically, mental health professionals can support school staff in monitoring students' SDoE and early signs of academic difficulty and school disengagement. Youth with such risk factors should be prioritized for increased social and emotional supports, with a focus on parental engagement and tailoring of the educational plan to align with the youth's interests, abilities, and culture. During transition periods, schools should bolster supports to encourage healthy development and prevention of substance use, gang involvement, and risky sexual behaviors. Importantly, it is incumbent on mental health clinicians to continue in antiracist self-education, reflection, and self-evaluation. Key areas for self-monitoring include the overuse of disruptive behavior diagnoses in youth of color, which can negatively affect both the perception of the child and the resources the school provides, and the assessment for underrecognized areas of concern such as anxiety, depressive, or trauma-related disorders.

SUMMARY

Because of complex and entrenched racial inequity in the US education system, Black, Latinx, American Indian, and other youth of color have disparate educational outcomes that are largely driven by SDoE, which include their community of residence, school funding, and burden of ACEs. The resulting educational disparities involve exclusionary systems of discipline and bias that lead to increased carceral contact and reduced educational achievement. Opportunities to improve educational disparities in minoritized youth include enacting antiracist policies, centering community partners, implementing whole-school trauma-informed approaches, and investing in antiracist classrooms. Mental health clinicians can contribute to these efforts by advocating for developmentally informed practices, lending a preventative lens, and reflecting on the equity of their diagnostic practices.

CLINICS CARE POINTS

- Racial disparities in the US education system are influenced by a long history of structural racism, not group differences between youth.
- Reducing teacher bias, clinician bias, and exclusionary discipline are prime targets for system transformation.
- Mental health clinicians can offer advocacy, a developmental framework, and trauma-informed practices.

DISCLOSURE

Drs E. Dohrmann, M.V. Porche, R. Ijadi-Maghsoodi, and S.H. Kataoka do not have any relationships with any commercial companies with direct financial interests related to the content of this article.

REFERENCES

1. Duong MT, Bruns EJ, Lee K, et al. Rates of mental health service utilization by children and adolescents in schools and other common service settings: a systematic review and meta-analysis. Adm Policy Ment Heal Ment Heal Serv Res 2021. https://doi.org/10.1007/s10488-020-01080-9.
2. Morris EW, Perry BL. The punishment gap: school suspension and racial disparities in achievement. Soc Probl 2016. https://doi.org/10.1093/socpro/spv026.
3. Coker TR, Elliott MN, Kanouse DE, et al. Perceived racial/ethnic discrimination among fifth-grade students and its association with mental health. Am J Public Health 2009. https://doi.org/10.2105/AJPH.2008.144329.
4. Fortuna LR, Tolou-Shams M, Robles-Ramamurthy B, et al. Inequity and the disproportionate impact of COVID-19 on communities of color in the United States: the need for a trauma-informed social justice response. Psychol Trauma 2020. https://doi.org/10.1037/tra0000889.
5. Bailey DH, Duncan GJ, Murnane RJ, et al. Achievement gaps in the wake of COVID-19. Educ Res 2021. https://doi.org/10.3102/0013189X211011237.
6. Hoffman JA, Miller EA. Addressing the consequences of school closure due to COVID-19 on children's physical and mental well-being. World Med Health Policy 2020. https://doi.org/10.1002/wmh3.365.
7. Ijadi-Maghsoodi R, Harrison D, Kelman A, et al. Leveraging a public-public partnership in los angeles county to address COVID-19 for children, youth, and families in underresourced communities. Psychol Trauma 2020. https://doi.org/10.1037/tra0000880.
8. Masonbrink AR, Hurley E. Advocating for children during the COVID-19 school closures. Pediatrics 2020. https://doi.org/10.1542/PEDS.2020-1440.
9. Rozenfeld Y, Beam J, Maier H, et al. A model of disparities: risk factors associated with COVID-19 infection. Int J Equity Health 2020. https://doi.org/10.1186/s12939-020-01242-z.
10. Maness SB, Merrell L, Thompson EL, et al. Social determinants of health and health disparities: COVID-19 exposures and mortality among African American people in the United States. Public Health Rep 2021. https://doi.org/10.1177/0033354920969169.
11. Krieger N. Embodying inequality: a review of concepts, measures, and methods for studying health consequences of discrimination. Int J Health Serv 1999. https://doi.org/10.2190/M11W-VWXE-KQM9-G97Q.
12. Ramirez M, Wu Y, Kataoka S, et al. Youth violence across multiple dimensions: a study of violence, absenteeism, and suspensions among middle school children. J Pediatr 2012. https://doi.org/10.1016/j.jpeds.2012.03.014.
13. Lacour M, Tissington LD. The effects of poverty on academic achievement. Educ Res Rev 2011.
14. Individuals with Disabilities Education Act, 20 U.S.C. § 1400 (2004).; 2004.
15. Suldo SM, Gormley MJ, DuPaul GJ, et al. The impact of school mental health on student and school-level academic outcomes: current status of the research and future directions. School Ment Health; 2014. https://doi.org/10.1007/s12310-013-9116-2.
16. Sotto-Santiago S. Time to reconsider the word minority in academic medicine. J Best Pr Heal Prof Divers 2019;12(1):72–8.
17. Sulkowski ML, Joyce-Beaulieu DK. School-based service delivery for homeless students: relevant laws and overcoming access barriers. Am J Orthopsychiatry 2014. https://doi.org/10.1037/ort0000033.

18. Rothstein R. The myth of de facto segregation. Phi Delta Kappan 2019. https://doi.org/10.1177/0031721719827543.

19. Ingram ES, Bridgeland JM, Reed B, et al. Hidden in plain sight: homeless students in America's public schools. Civ Enterp 2017.

20. Croninger RG, Lee VE. Social capital and dropping out of high school: benefits to at-risk students of teachers' support and guidance. Teach Coll Rec 2001. https://doi.org/10.1111/0161-4681.00127.

21. Fadus MC, Ginsburg KR, Sobowale K, et al. Unconscious bias and the diagnosis of disruptive behavior disorders and ADHD in African American and hispanic youth. Acad Psychiatry 2020. https://doi.org/10.1007/s40596-019-01127-6.

22. Porche MV, Fortuna LR, Lin J, et al. Childhood trauma and psychiatric disorders as correlates of school dropout in a national sample of young adults. Child Dev 2011. https://doi.org/10.1111/j.1467-8624.2010.01534.x.

23. Hussar B, Zhang J, Hein S, Wang K, Roberts A, Mary JC. The Condition of Education 2020 (NCES 2020-144).; 2020.

24. Alegria M, Vallas M, Pumariega AJ. Racial and ethnic disparities in pediatric mental health. Child Adolesc Psychiatr Clin N Am 2010. https://doi.org/10.1016/j.chc.2010.07.001.

25. Woods-Jaeger BA, Hampton-Anderson J, Christensen K, et al. School-based racial microaggressions: a barrier to resilience among African American adolescents exposed to trauma. Psychol Trauma 2021. https://doi.org/10.1037/tra0001091.

26. Noltemeyer AL. The history of inequality in education. Disporportionality Educ Spec Educ 2012.

27. Plessy vs. Ferguson, Judgement, Decided May 18, 1896; Records of the Supreme Court of the United States; Record Group 267; Plessy v. Ferguson, 163, #15248, National Archives.

28. Ovington MW. The National Association for the advancement of colored people. J Negro Hist 1924. https://doi.org/10.2307/2713634.

29. Warren, E. & Supreme Court Of The United States. (1953) U.S. Reports: Brown v. Board of Education, 347 U.S. 483.

30. Brown F. The first serious implementation of brown: the 1964 civil rights act and beyond. J Negro Educ 2004. https://doi.org/10.2307/4129604.

31. Kelly H. Race, Remembering, and Jim Crow's Teachers.; 2010. doi:10.4324/9780203852354

32. Bristol TJ, Martin-Fernandez J. The added value of latinx and black teachers for latinx and black students: implications for policy. Policy Insights Behav Brain Sci 2019. https://doi.org/10.1177/2372732219862573.

33. Kantor H. Education, social reform, and the state: ESEA and federal education policy in the 1960s. Am J Educ 1991. https://doi.org/10.1086/444004.

34. Orfield G, Lee C. Historic reversals, accelerating resegregation, and the need for new integration strategies. Civ Rights Proj; 2007.

35. Callet VJ. Test review: high-stakes testing: does the California high school exit exam measure up? Lang Assess Q 2005. https://doi.org/10.1207/s15434311laq0204_3.

36. Black DW. Abandoning the federal role in education: the every student Succeeds act. Calif Law Rev 2017. https://doi.org/10.15779/Z38Z31NN9K.

37. George J. Populating the pipeline: school policing and the persistence of the school-to-prison pipeline. Nova Law Rev 2016;40(3):6.

38. Allen Q, White-Smith KA. "Just as bad as prisons": the challenge of dismantling the school-to-prison pipeline through teacher and community education. Equity Excell Educ 2014. https://doi.org/10.1080/10665684.2014.958961.
39. Counts J, Randall KN, Ryan JB, et al. School resource officers in public schools: a national review. Educ Treat Child 2018. https://doi.org/10.1353/etc.2018.0023.
40. Gottlieb A, Wilson R. The effect of direct and vicarious police contact on the educational achievement of urban teens. Child Youth Serv Rev 2019. https://doi.org/10.1016/j.childyouth.2019.06.009.
41. Wallace JM, Goodkind S, Wallace CM, et al. Racial, ethnic, and gender differences in school discipline among U.S. High school students: 1991-2005. Negro Educ Rev 2008.
42. Harry B, Klingner J. Discarding the deficit model. Educ Leadersh 2007.
43. Banks T. From deficit to divergence: refocusing special education for African Americans labeled as having emotional and behavioral problems. In: Special Education Practices: Personal Narratives of African American Scholars, Educators, and Related Professionals. ; 2012.
44. Gregory A, Skiba RJ, Noguera PA. The achievement gap and the discipline gap: two sides of the same coin? Educ Res 2010. https://doi.org/10.3102/0013189X09357621.
45. Muhammad F. African American resilience: the need for policy in escaping the trap of special education. Urban Educ Res Policy Annu 2016;4(1):138–46.
46. Fish RE. Standing out and sorting in: exploring the role of racial composition in racial disparities in special education. Am Educ Res J 2019. https://doi.org/10.3102/0002831219847966.
47. Grindal T, Schifter LA, Schwartz G, et al. Racial differences in special education identification and placement: evidence across three states. Harv Educ Rev 2019. https://doi.org/10.17763/1943-5045-89.4.525.
48. Chin MJ, Quinn DM, Dhaliwal TK, et al. Bias in the air: a nationwide exploration of teachers' implicit racial attitudes, aggregate bias, and student outcomes. Educ Res 2020. https://doi.org/10.3102/0013189X20937240.
49. Meléndez Guevara AM, White RMB, Lindstrom Johnson S, et al. School racial-ethnic discrimination, rule-breaking behaviors and the mediating role of trauma among latinx adolescents: considerations for school mental health practice. Psychol Sch 2021. https://doi.org/10.1002/pits.22562.
50. Grossman JM, Porche MV. Perceived gender and racial/ethnic barriers to STEM success. Urban Educ 2014. https://doi.org/10.1177/0042085913481364.
51. Gilliam WS. Prekindergarteners Left behind: Expulsion Rates in State Prekindergarten Systems.; 2005.
52. Rights O for C. Civil rights data collection. Available at: https://ocrdata.ed.gov/estimations/2017-2018.
53. Skiba RJ, Michael RS, Nardo AC, et al. The color of discipline: sources of racial and gender disproportionality in school punishment. Urban Rev 2002. https://doi.org/10.1023/A:1021320817372.
54. Choi KR, O'Malley C, Ijadi-Maghsoodi R, Tascione E, Bath E, Zima BT. A Scoping Review of Police Involvement in School Crisis Response for Mental Health Emergencies _ Enhanced Reader.pdf. 2021.
55. Fisher BW, Hennessy EA. School resource officers and exclusionary discipline in U.S. high schools: a systematic review and meta-analysis. Adolesc Res Rev 2016. https://doi.org/10.1007/s40894-015-0006-8.
56. Felitti VJ, Anda RF, Nordenberg D, et al. Relationship of childhood abuse and household dysfunction to many of the leading causes of death in adults: the

adverse childhood experiences (ACE) study. Am J Prev Med 1998. https://doi.org/10.1016/S0749-3797(98)00017-8.

57. Baglivio M, Epps N, Swartz K, et al. The prevalence of adverse childhood experiences (ACE) in the lives of juvenile offenders. J Juv Justice 2013.

58. Crouch JL, Hanson RF, Saunders BE, et al. Income, race/ethnicity, and exposure to violence in youth: results from the national survey of adolescents. J Community Psychol 2000. https://doi.org/10.1002/1520-6629(200011)28:6<625::AID-JCOP6>3.0.CO;2-R.

59. Mikolajewski AJ, Scheeringa MS. Links between oppositional defiant disorder dimensions, psychophysiology, and interpersonal versus non-interpersonal trauma. J Psychopathol Behav Assess 2021. https://doi.org/10.1007/s10862-021-09930-y.

60. Beltrán S, Sit L, Ginsburg KR. A call to revise the diagnosis of oppositional defiant disorder - diagnoses are for helping, not harming. JAMA Psychiatry 2021. https://doi.org/10.1001/jamapsychiatry.2021.2127.

61. Feisthamel K, Schwartz R. Differences in mental health counselors' diagnoses based on client race: an investigation of adjustment, childhood, and substance-related disorders. J Ment Health Couns 2009. https://doi.org/10.17744/mehc.31.1.u82021637276wv1k.

62. Grimmett MA, Dunbar AS, Williams T, et al. The process and implications of diagnosing oppositional defiant disorder in African American Males. Prof Couns 2016. https://doi.org/10.15241/mg.6.2.147.

63. DeFosset AR, Gase LN, Ijadi-Maghsoodi R, et al. Youth descriptions of mental health needs and experiences with school- based services: identifying ways to meet the needs of underserved adolescents. J Health Care Poor Underserved 2017. https://doi.org/10.1353/hpu.2017.0105.

64. Ijadi-Maghsoodi R, Venegas-Murillo A, Klomhaus A, et al. The role of resilience and gender: understanding the relationship between risk for traumatic stress, resilience, and academic outcomes among minoritized youth. Psychol Trauma 2022. https://doi.org/10.1037/tra0001161. Online ahead of print.

65. Spencer AE, Sikov J, Loubeau JK, et al. Six stages of engagement in ADHD treatment described by diverse, urban parents. Pediatrics 2021. https://doi.org/10.1542/peds.2021-051261.

66. Ward C. Theories of justice underpinning equity in education for refugee and asylum-seeking youth in the U.S.: considering Rawls, Sandel, and Sen. Ethics Educ 2020. https://doi.org/10.1080/17449642.2020.1774721.

67. Knoester M, Au W. Standardized testing and school segregation: like tinder for fire? Race Ethn Educ 2017. https://doi.org/10.1080/13613324.2015.1121474.

68. Congressional report service. 2018. Available at: https://crsreports.congress.gov/product/pdf/R/R45251.

69. King M, Perkins ER. Discipline foundation policy: school-wide positive behavior intervention and support. Available at: https://achieve.lausd.net/site/handlers/filedownload.ashx?moduleinstanceid=23778&dataid=25844&FileName=BUL-6231.0 DISCIPLINE FOUNDATION POLICY.pdf.

70. Board of education of the City of Los Angeles: special meeting order of business. 2021. Available at: http://laschoolboard.org/sites/default/files/02-16-21SpclBdOBWithMaterialsColor.pdf.

71. Maier A, Daniel J, Oakes J, et al. Community schools as an effective school improvement strategy: a Review of the evidence. Learn Policy Inst. 2017;(December):1-159. Available at: https://learningpolicyinstitute.org/product/

%0Ahttps://learningpolicyinstitute.org/sites/default/files/product-files/Community_Schools_Effective_REPORT.pdf.

72. Fallon LM, Veiga M, Sugai G. Strengthening MTSS for behavior (MTSS-B) to promote racial equity. School Psych Rev 2021. https://doi.org/10.1080/2372966X.2021.1972333.

73. Braithwaite J. Restorative Justice : Theories and Worries. 123Rd Int Sr Semin Visit Expert Pap. 1989.

74. Augustine C, Engberg J, Grimm G, et al. Can Restorative Practices Improve School Climate and Curb Suspensions? An Evaluation of the Impact of Restorative Practices in a Mid-Sized Urban School District.; 2019. doi:10.7249/rr2840

75. Darling-Hammond S, Fronius TA, Sutherland H, et al. Effectiveness of restorative justice in US K-12 schools: a review of quantitative research. Contemp Sch Psychol 2020. https://doi.org/10.1007/s40688-020-00290-0.

76. Blitz LV, Anderson EM, Saastamoinen M. Assessing perceptions of culture and trauma in an elementary school: informing a model for culturally responsive trauma-informed schools. Urban Rev 2016. https://doi.org/10.1007/s11256-016-0366-9.

77. Koslouski JB, Stark K. Promoting learning for students experiencing adversity and trauma: the everyday, yet profound, actions of teachers. Elem Sch J 2021. https://doi.org/10.1086/712606.

78. Joseph AA, Wilcox SM, Hnilica RJ, et al. Keeping race at the center of school discipline practices and trauma-informed care: an interprofessional framework. Child Sch 2020. https://doi.org/10.1093/cs/cdaa013.

79. Bassok D, Galdo E. Inequality in preschool quality? Community-level disparities in access to high-quality learning environments. Early Educ Dev 2016. https://doi.org/10.1080/10409289.2015.1057463.

80. Latham S, Corcoran SP, Sattin-Bajaj C, et al. Racial disparities in Pre-K quality: evidence from New York City's Universal Pre-K Program. Educ Res 2021. https://doi.org/10.3102/0013189x211028214.

81. Schweinhart LJ. Long-term follow-up of a preschool experiment. J Exp Criminol 2013. https://doi.org/10.1007/s11292-013-9190-3.

82. Davis AE, Perry DF, Rabinovitz L. Expulsion prevention: framework for the role of infant and early childhood mental health consultation in addressing implicit biases. Infant Ment Health J 2020. https://doi.org/10.1002/imhj.21847.

83. Yull D, Wilson M, Murray C, Parham L. Reversing the dehumanization of families of color in schools: community-based research in a race-conscious parent engagement program. Sch community J 2018.

84. Li A, Fischer MJ. Advantaged/disadvantaged school neighborhoods, parental networks, and parental involvement at elementary school. Sociol Educ 2017. https://doi.org/10.1177/0038040717732332.

85. Snyder FJ, Acock AC, Vuchinich S, et al. Preventing negative behaviors among elementary-school students through enhancing students' social-emotional and character development. Am J Health Promot 2013. https://doi.org/10.4278/ajhp.120419-QUAN-207.2.

86. Jeynes WH. A meta-analysis of the relation of parental involvement to urban elementary school student academic achievement. Urban Educ 2005. https://doi.org/10.1177/0042085905274540.

87. Nansel TR, Haynie DL, Simonsmorton BG. The association of bullying and victimization with middle school adjustment. J Appl Sch Psychol 2003. https://doi.org/10.1300/J008v19n02_04.

88. Hong JS, Peguero AA, Espelage DL. Experiences in bullying and/or peer victimization of vulnerable, marginalized, and oppressed children and adolescents: an introduction to the special issue. Am J Orthopsychiatry 2018. https://doi.org/10.1037/ort0000330.

89. Schneider B, Martinez S, Owens A. Barriers to educational opportunities for hispanics in the United States. In: Hispanics and the future of America. ; 2006. doi:10.17226/11539

90. Olweus D, Limber SP, Breivik K. Addressing specific forms of bullying: a large-scale evaluation of the olweus bullying prevention program. Int J Bullying Prev 2019. https://doi.org/10.1007/s42380-019-00009-7.

91. Williams MT, Metzger IW, Leins C, et al. Assessing racial trauma within a DSM–5 framework: the UConn racial/ethnic stress & trauma survey. Pract Innov 2018. https://doi.org/10.1037/pri0000076.

92. Williams MT, Printz DMB, DeLapp RCT. Assessing racial trauma with the trauma symptoms of discrimination scale. Psychol Violence 2018. https://doi.org/10.1037/vio0000212s.

Suicide and Suicidal Behaviors Among Minoritized Youth

Tami D. Benton, MD[a,b]

KEYWORDS

- Suicidality • Asian American/Pacific Islander • Hispanic • Black • Pediatric
- Adolescent • Disparities

KEY POINTS

- Suicide is among the leading causes of death for American Indian/Alaskan Native, Asian American/Pacific Islanders, black, Hispanic, and multiracial youth. Although recent data suggest increasing trends in suicide and suicidal behaviors among minoritized populations, limited research is available to understand these trends. Emerging data regarding suicidal ideation, attempts, and suicide deaths suggest increasing trends among minoritized populations. Youth who identify as racial/ethnic minorities and sexual minorities appear to be at even greater risk. Existing data suggest a disparity in recognition and interventions for these vulnerable populations.
- Trends in suicidal ideation and behaviors for minoritized youth populations show some variations in age of onset, gender disparities, and outcomes when compared with white youth.
- Interventions targeting suicide and suicidal behaviors among diverse youth are lacking, calling for increased research support for understanding this growing population of youth.

INTRODUCTION

Suicide and suicidal behaviors continue to be a significant public health problem.[1–4] It remains the second leading cause of death for youth aged 10 to 24 years, taking more young lives than all medical disorders of childhood combined.[1] Emerging data further suggest worsening trends in suicidal behaviors since the onset of COVID-19. During February 21 to March 20, 2021, emergency department visits for suspected suicide attempts were 50.6% higher among girls aged 12 to 17 years than during the same time period in the prior year, whereas for boys, suspected suicide attempts increased by 3.7%. In some states and jurisdictions, suicide has become the leading cause of death.[5]

[a] Department of Child and Adolescent Psychiatry and Behavioral Sciences, Children's Hospital of Philadelphia, 3440 Market Street, Suite 400, Philadelphia, PA 19104, USA; [b] Perelman School of Medicine, University of Pennsylvania, Philadelphia, PA, USA
E-mail address: BENTONT@chop.edu

Child Adolesc Psychiatric Clin N Am 31 (2022) 211–221
https://doi.org/10.1016/j.chc.2022.01.002
1056-4993/22/Published by Elsevier Inc.

childpsych.theclinics.com

Suicide and suicidal behaviors are complex phenomena without a single cause, complicating efforts to predict who will make a suicide attempt or die by suicide. Although rates of completed suicide among children and adolescents are very low, 2.57/100,000 adolescents aged 10 to 14 years and 10.5/100,000 adolescents aged 15 to 19 years,[1] suicide attempts occur at a much higher rate and are associated with significant morbidity.[1,6,7]

Most recent data examining suicide and suicidal behaviors among youth have been obtained through the Youth Risk Behavior Surveillance System, a school-based survey for ninth through twelfth graders that is collected every 2 years by the Centers for Disease Control and Prevention asking adolescents about health behaviors they have experienced in the 12 months before the survey. The data collected represent a national sample of youth from US states, territorial, and tribal governments. Approximately 30 years of cross-sectional data have been collected reflecting trends in suicide and suicidal behaviors for 1991 to 2019. Findings from the most recent nationwide Youth Risk Behavior Survey completed in 2019 found that 16% of all high school students (grades 9–12) reported suicidal thoughts with a plan in the past year; 9% had made a suicide attempt, and 3% of attempters required medical intervention. These most recent data also found significant differences in rates of these behaviors among ethnic/racial minorities and lesbian, gay, bisexual, transgender, and queer (LGBTQ)+ youth.

Historically, rates of suicide and suicidal behaviors have been reported to be low among minoritized youth, which includes African American (AA)/black, American Indian/Alaskan Native (AI/AN), Asian American/Pacific Island/Native Hawaiians (AAPI), Hispanic, and multiracial youth, with the exception of Native American/Alaskan Native youth.[1] Consequently, little research has focused on minoritized youth, with the assumption that suicide was most relevant in white youth. However, recent research has challenged these assumptions and is beginning to identify trends in suicide and suicidal behaviors among minoritized populations, noting variations in suicidal behaviors that appear to be specific to these groups. For example, trends in suicidal ideation and behaviors increase with age across childhood and adolescence; however, variations in age of onset of suicidality have been noted in Native American and black youth with earlier age of onset found for Native American and black boys.[8] Disparities in suicide rates have also been found among black boys with rates of suicide increasing for 5- to 11-year-olds while at the same time declining for same-aged white boys.

This review focuses on trends in suicide and suicidal behavior observed among AA/black, AI/AN, Asian American/Pacific Island Hispanic, and multiracial youth, recent evidence-based and promising interventions for suicidal ideation, and behaviors for children and adolescents, emerging studies of culturally adapted suicide interventions for minoritized youth and directions for future research.

AFRICAN AMERICAN/BLACK YOUTH

Published studies of youth suicide research in the United States have reported lower rates of suicide and suicidal behavior (suicidal ideation and behaviors [SIB]) for black youth compared with other racial and ethnic groups. Emerging research, however, raises questions about prior research reporting lower rates and concerns about racial disparities.[2] For AA/black youth, rates of suicide have been increasing over the last 10 years.[8–10]

In 2019, suicide was the third leading cause of death for AA/black youth aged 5 to 19 years (3.12/100,000), a significant increase compared with rates reported in 2009 (1.98/100,000). Overall, a 58% increase in suicide rates for AA/black youth was observed between 2009 and 2019. For black youth aged 10 to 14 years of age, a 131.5% increase was observed between 1999 and 2019. The gender disparities noted in other populations were not the same as those observed in AA/black youth. Boys and girls aged 5 to 17 years experienced increased suicide rates between 2003 and 2017, with suicide rates for black girls showing twice the annual percentage change compared with black boys.[3] Across age groups, suicide rates were highest for girls and boys aged 15 through 17 years.[3]

Several studies examining suicidal ideation and attempts for black youth have reported similar findings.[2] Youth Risk Behavior Survey (YRBS) data from 1991 to 2017 found that black adolescents experienced not only a significant increase in suicide attempts but also suicide attempts that required medical attention. Price and Khubchandani reviewed suicide trends among AA/black adolescents from 2001 to 2017, finding a significant increase in suicidal ideation, plans, and attempts requiring medical treatment.[11] Interestingly, the data also showed that black youth were more likely to make suicide attempts, but were less likely to report suicidal ideation or plans.[12] YRBS data analyzed from 2009 through 2019 confirmed a significant increase in rates of attempted suicide among black youth.[10] Bridge and colleagues, in a study of suicide rates using psychological autopsy data of 5- to 12-year-old black children, found that black children were 2 times more likely to die than same-aged white youth, suggesting an age disparity for black youth, with suicide for black youth occurring at earlier ages.[8]

Recent reports of increasing rates of black youth suicide prompted Representative Bonnie Coleman-Watson to convene a multidisciplinary task force of the congressional black caucus to study black youth suicide with the goal of improved identification, intervention, and prevention, prompting increased research focus to understand risks, resilience, and protective factors for suicide in the black youth population.[13]

AMERICAN INDIAN/ALASKAN NATIVE YOUTH

Suicide is the leading cause of death for AI/AN youth aged 15 to 19 years of age and the second leading cause of death among youth aged 10 to 14 years. Rates of completed suicide are notably high among AI/AN youth with suicide death 3 times higher than overall rates of suicide deaths among children and adolescents in the United States.

AI/AN youth aged 10 to 19 years have the highest rates of completed suicide across all racial and ethnic populations for boys (18.83/100,000) and girls (8.79/100,000). Gender differences have been observed for AI/AN girls having increased prevalence of suicidal ideation compared with other racial/ethnic groups with AI/AN boys showing higher rates of suicide attempts. The most recent YRBS surveys found that AI/AN youth were more likely to endorse suicidal ideation (1.43 times more) and to report a suicide attempt (1.46 times) in the 12 months before the survey compared with white youth.[14]

Other studies examining suicidal ideation and behaviors among AI/AN youth have sought to understand factors influencing rates of SIB. Manzo and colleagues reviewed YRBS data covering 2005 to 2011 for AI/AN students attending urban schools compared with those attending tribal schools.[15] Rates of suicidal ideation (SI) were higher for youth attending urban schools compared with those attending tribal schools. Similar findings were identified for suicide attempts among AI/AN youth. Gender differences were noted, however, with AI/AN girls attending urban schools reporting similar prevalence of suicide attempts compared with tribal schools, whereas boys in urban schools reported higher prevalence of suicide attempt (SA) compared with tribal schools, suggesting that a culturally concordant environment may play some role as a protective factor for boys.[15]

ASIAN AMERICAN, PACIFIC ISLANDER, AND NATIVE HAWAIIAN YOUTH

Suicide is the leading cause of death for AAPI youth aged 10 to 19 years of age. It is the number one cause of death for 10- to 19-year-olds and 15- to 19-year-olds, and the third leading cause of death for 10- to 14-year-olds.[16]

Despite an increase in suicide deaths by 131.8% occurring between 2009 and 2019 for AAPI youth, very little data exist examining these trends, risk factors, or circumstances influencing these high suicide rates. Several analyses of YRBS data have shed little light on suicide and suicidal behaviors among AAPI youth. For example, one analysis of data from 1991 to 2017 found decreased suicidal ideation and behaviors.[2] Another study examining suicidality among AAPI youth found significant decreases in suicide plans and behavior but no decrease in suicidal ideation or attempts.[17] In some studies, gender differences were studied and have been noted among AAPI youth; however, the observed differences reflected differing temporal trends with declines in suicidal ideation for girls observed between 1991 and 2019 and decreasing SI noted for boys between 1991 and 2006, making comparisons difficult.

Other studies attempting to understand trends and risks for SIB for AAPI youth have examined suicide attempts by racial/ethnic group status. One study used the Native Hawaiian High School Health Survey for this purpose. The study's findings were that Native Hawaiians reported significantly higher rates of suicide attempts compared with white, Filipino, and Japanese adolescents.[18] Another school-based study found that adolescents exposed to violence at school were more likely to have suicidal plans and a history of attempts.[19] Currently, the limited data available focused on suicide and suicidal behaviors in the AAPI population prevent formulations about suicide trends among AAPI youth, calling for increased support for studying suicide in AAPI populations.

HISPANIC YOUTH

Suicide is the second leading cause of death for Hispanic youth aged 15 to 19 years, and the third leading cause of death among 10- to 14-year-olds.[16] Suicide continues to trend upwards significantly for Hispanic adolescents, with notable increases observed for early adolescents. Between 2015 and 2019, suicide deaths increased by 89% among boys aged 10 to 14 years and by 79% for girls. Among youth aged 15 to 19 years, suicide-related death rates increased by 29% among boys but remained stable among girls. From 2007 to 2016, the ratio of male-to-female suicide deaths for youth aged 10 to 19 years decreased, driven by the increased numbers of suicide deaths for Hispanic girls.[20] Between 1991 and 2019, rates of suicidal ideation were relatively stable for Hispanic girls and boys, whereas suicide attempts showed a downward trend. Although downward trends were noted for suicide attempts among Hispanic girls from 1991 to 2009, rates began to increase from 2009 to 2019. Rates for Hispanic boys did not change across this time period.[20]

Recently, studies have increasingly focused on contextual factors, systemic and structural, impacting Hispanic youth that might contribute to SIB. One structural factor significantly impacting these youth are current immigration policies, with one recent study finding that 25% of Hispanic adolescents surveyed had a family member who had been detained or deported in the past year. This finding was associated with 2.63 greater odds of SI compared with nonimmigrant peers. Contextual factors must be considered when examining suicide risks for minoritized and vulnerable youth.[21]

MULTIRACIAL YOUTH

Even more limited data exist regarding suicide deaths and suicidal behaviors for multiracial youth. Several factors contribute to the limited knowledge of this group. Early data collection efforts were hampered by low numbers of self-identified multiracial individuals. Furthermore, heterogeneity in group composition makes it difficult to identify a "target group." However, the existing data reflecting trends in suicidality among multiracial youth raise cause for concern. Recent data from the YRBS found higher prevalence of suicidal ideation (26.2%), suicide plans (20.7%), and suicide attempts (13%) in comparison to rates for white youths (18.9%, 14.4%, and 6.7%). The study also found an association between alcohol and tobacco use and suicidal ideation, plans, and attempts for multiracial groups.[14]

Multiracial youth are one of the fastest growing populations of youth in the United States, yet little is known about suicide risks for this population. A recent published study examining trends in suicidal behaviors from 1991 to 2017 using the YRBS data found no significant changes in suicide attempts, suicidal ideation, or plans for multiracial high school students. However, the limited research available does not allow for conclusions, calling for increased focus on this population of youth. Given the rapid growth of this population, increased focus is imperative.[22]

Across ethnic and racial groups, higher rates of suicide and suicidal behaviors have been reported for LGBTQ+ youth of color compared with white LGBTQ+ youth. This growing population of youth identifying as sexual and racial/ethnic minorities is an at-risk group requiring significant research focus.[17,23–25]

ASSESSMENT OF SUICIDE FOR YOUTH: RACISM AND RACIAL TRAUMA

As previously noted, suicide is influenced by multiple interacting factors. The biopsychosocial model posits that genetic, experiential, psychological, clinical, sociologic, and environmental factors contribute to an individual's suicide risk. A comprehensive review of suicide assessment can be found in an excellent review by Turecki and colleagues[6]. Any or all of these factors may interact at a given time to precipitate suicidality for an individual; however, their relative contributions to risk for suicide will be mediated by factors unique to that individual. For example, depression is commonly present among those who have attempted and died by suicide; however, the presence of depression among those with suicidal ideation does not inevitably lead to a suicide attempt or death. Depression and its proximal association with a suicide attempt is mediated by other factors that make suicide a more likely outcome. The elevated rates of SIB identified among minoritized youth populations must be considered within the context of racism, racial trauma, and xenophobia and should be assessed as an integral component of the conceptual framework when evaluating youth. The negative impact of racial stress and trauma, identified as an adverse childhood experience, has been well documented.[26] These factors, racism and discrimination, must be considered in the mental health assessments of minoritized youth when assessing causes for suicidal behaviors, developing treatment plans, and interventions. For example, some studies suggest improved treatment outcomes with cultural adapted interventions or racially concordant therapists.[27–31] A recent meta-analysis found that therapy with a majority of black youth had lower effect sizes when youth lived in states with greater anti-black racism compared with states with less anti-black racism, demonstrating the effects of racism on treatment outcomes for minoritized youth.[32]

TREATMENTS FOR SUICIDAL YOUTH OF COLOR

As with all suicidal youth, a comprehensive assessment for underlying psychiatric conditions should inform selected interventions. Depression, substance use, or other psychiatric disorders should be identified and treated with evidence-supported interventions, including pharmacotherapy and psychotherapy when indicated. Fortunately, increased focus on suicide prevention for adolescents and young adults has produced effective psychotherapeutic interventions. Some of the intervention trials have included minoritized youth populations in their studies, with most reporting limited representation; thus, these interventions are not well studied for minoritized youth populations. Interventions available for suicidal youth consist of individually focused interventions, family-focused interventions, and multicomponent interventions, which are discussed later. Recent reviews report that dialectical behavior therapy for adolescents (DBT-A) is the only intervention meeting criteria as a well-established treatment for reducing suicidal ideation and behavior in adolescents, but others are promising.[33]

INDIVIDUALLY FOCUSED INTERVENTIONS
Dialectical Behavior Therapy for Adolescents

DBT-A is a multicomponent cognitive-behavioral treatment that targets emotional, interpersonal, and behavioral dysregulation that leads to self-injurious thoughts and behaviors.[34] DBT-A has been found to be an effective clinical intervention for adolescents presenting with self-injurious thoughts and behaviors.[35] In an randomized controlled trial (RCT), adolescents with a history of deliberate self-harm and borderline personality disordered features receiving a shortened form of DBT-A (19 weeks vs typical 6-month package) showed significantly greater reductions in deliberate self-harm and suicidal ideation over the course of treatment and at the end of the 19 weeks than adolescents in enhanced usual care (weekly psychodynamic or cognitive-behavioral therapy, plus medication as usual).[36] A second RCT compared DBT-A with individual and group supportive therapy in a sample of adolescents with a history of suicide attempts and found that the adolescents receiving DBT-A reported significantly fewer instances of deliberate self-harm, nonsuicidal self-injury, and suicidal behavior as well as reductions in suicidal ideation from baseline to 6 months.[33]

DBT-A itself consists of multiple components: individual therapy, skills training group, phone coaching, and ancillary treatment. The skills training group is primarily focused on teaching skills for enhancing emotion regulation in addition to other constructs, such as distress tolerance and interpersonal effectiveness. In addition, keeping in mind the research demonstrating the efficacy of family components in interventions targeting adolescent suicidality, the skills training group adapted for DBT-A is multifamily, consisting of a group of adolescents and their parents. According to DBT theory, the behaviors of suicidal and self-injurious individuals stem from a combination of a biological sensitivity and environmental factors.[34]

Cognitive behavioral therapy (CBT) for suicide prevention (CBT-SP)[35] developed from a recognition that traditional CBT for depression does not adequately address suicidality. CBT-SP as designed for adolescents integrates traditional components of CBT for depression, such as cognitive restructuring and behavioral activation, with elements of DBT-A. In addition, there is an emphasis on family engagement and collaboration, an important addition given the role of family factors in the development of suicidality. CBT-SP aims to target suicidal feelings through teaching several different emotion regulation skills, including relaxation, mindfulness, emotion identification, and hope building. The overall goal of this treatment is to reduce the risk of suicidal behaviors in adolescents.

Interpersonal psychotherapy for adolescents (IPT-A) is another individually focused therapeutic intervention that has shown promise in the treatment of youth presenting with self-injurious thoughts and behaviors. School-based IPT-A significantly reduced suicidal ideation compared with treatment as usual (ie, psychoeducation and supportive counseling).[37,38] Although IPT-A focuses on the impact of adolescents' interpersonal relationships on psychiatric symptoms and overall functioning, there is also an emphasis on emotion education and awareness, mood monitoring, and feeling expression.

FAMILY-FOCUSED INTERVENTIONS FOR SUICIDE

It is not surprising that several psychosocial interventions for suicide target family context factors directly or include a component focused on family relationships.[39] For example, Attachment-Based Family Therapy (ABFT), which is rooted in attachment theory, teaches interpersonal and affect regulation skills with the goal of improving the quality of parent-adolescent relationships and fostering a sense of relational security in which the adolescent can confront and manage difficult issues.[40] In an RCT, adolescents in ABFT showed significantly greater improvements in suicidal ideation than adolescents in enhanced usual care.[41] In a follow-up RCT comparing ABFT with family-enhanced nondirective supportive therapy (FE-NST), adolescents in ABFT showed significant reductions in suicidal ideation, but this change was not significantly different from the FE-NST comparison group.[42] ABFT is one of the few studies to include a racially diverse population.

Another example of a family-focused intervention is Safe Alternatives for Teens and Youths (SAFETY), a cognitive-behavioral family treatment that is informed by DBT and designed to prevent suicide attempts. SAFETY aims to bolster protective interpersonal supports within the family and teach skills that promote safer behaviors and reactions in the face of stressors. SAFETY has been shown to reduce suicidal ideation and prevent suicide attempts among high-risk youth.[43,44] Across studies, reviews of interventions for youth suicidal behaviors, investigators have concluded that those interventions that include a family component show the strongest evidence of efficacy in the treatment of suicidality and self-harm.[35,45,46] Thus, the evidence strongly suggests that a consideration of family context is an essential feature of interventions aimed at treatment of youth suicidality.

Although many more studies are focusing on suicide prevention for adolescents, few interventions have focused specifically on minoritized youth. However, burgeoning research has focused on AA, AAPI, NA/AI, and Hispanic youth. Three recent studies of culturally focused interventions are promising. A sociocognitive behavioral intervention was developed for SIB in Puerto Rican adolescents.[47] A school-based prevention program, including a cultural adapted-coping with stress course (A-CWS), has been developed for black youth at risk for suicide.[48] Another prevention program focused on AI/AN was implemented by community elders in junior high schools using a curricula focused on cultural values.[49] Much more research is needed to gain understanding of risk, resilience, and protective factors that will be needed to develop effective interventions that will be culturally acceptable.

SUMMARY

Suicide and suicidal behaviors are increasingly prevalent across all racial and ethnic groups, especially for youth identifying as racial/ethnic and sexual minorities. Currently, existing suicide research does not address prevention, identification, or interventions for these vulnerable populations. The tools that are used for screening, intervention, and prevention have demonstrated effectiveness for white youth, but have not been well studied for minoritized youth populations. It is unclear which factors contribute to the increasing rates of suicide and suicidal behaviors observed for youth of color. Although there are likely to be many similarities, there are also likely to be many differences within groups, such as multiracial groups, and between groups with different ethnic histories. However, there is one pressing need that is similar for all groups: there is a need for culturally appropriate interventions integrating contextual factors, including racism, racial trauma, xenophobia, and biases impacting minoritized youth. Increasing research that will support developing culturally appropriate, evidence-based interventions, and training the workforce to use them, will be required to stem the rising tide of suicide that we are observing among minoritized youth.

DISCLOSURE

Youth Suicide Prevention, Intervention and Research Center Deneen-Coyle fund is the source of funding.

REFERENCES

1. Centers for Disease Control and Prevention. Youth risk behavior survey data. Center for Disease Control and Prevention. 2019. Available at: www.cdc.gov/yrbs. Accessed September 02, 2021.
2. Lindsey MA, Sheftall AH, Xiao Y, et al. Trends of suicidal behaviors among high school students in the United States: 1991–2017. Pediatrics 2019;144(5): e20191187.
3. Sheftall AH, Vakil F, Ruch DA, et al. Black youth suicide: investigation of current trends and precipitating circumstances. J Am Acad Child Adolesc Psychiatry 2021. https://doi.org/10.1016/j.jaac.2021.08.021.
4. Yard E, Radhakrishnan L, Ballesteros MF, et al. Emergency department visits for suspected suicide attempts among persons aged 12–25 years before and during the COVID-19 pandemic — United States, January 2019–May 2021. MMWR Morb Mortal Wkly Rep 2021;70:888–94.
5. Children's Hospital Colorado declares a 'state of emergency' for youth mental health. childrenscolorado.org. 2021. Available at: https://www.childrenscolorado.org/about/news/2021/may-2021/youth-mental-health-state-of-emergency/. Accessed December 15, 2021.
6. Turecki G, Brent DA, Gunnell D, et al. Suicide and suicide risk. Nat Rev Dis Primers 2019;5(1):74.
7. National Center for Health Statistics. Underlying cause of death, 1999–2013. CDC WONDER online database. 2015. Available at: http://wonder.cdc.gov/ucd-icd10.html. Accessed December 20, 2021.
8. Bridge JA, Horowitz LM, Fontanella CA, et al. Age-related racial disparity in suicide rates among US youths from 2001 through 2015. JAMA Pediatr 2018;172(7): 697–9.
9. Bridge JA, Asti L, Horowitz LM, et al. Suicide trends among elementary school-aged children in the United States from 1993 to 2012. JAMA Pediatr. 2015; 169(7):673–7.
10. Ivey-Stephenson AZ, Demissie Z, Crosby AE, et al. Suicidal ideation and behaviors among high school students - youth risk behavior survey, United States, 2019. MMWR Suppl 2020;69(1):47–55.
11. Price JH, Khubchandani J. The changing characteristics of African-American adolescent suicides, 2001-2017. J Community Health 2019;44(4):756–63.

12. Romanelli M, Sheftall AH, Irsheid SB, et al. Factors associated with distinct patterns of suicidal thoughts, suicide plans, and suicide attempts among US adolescents. Prev Sci 2021;1–12. https://doi.org/10.1007/s11121-021-01295-8.
13. sprcnews.org. The Congressional Black Caucus Emergency Task Force. Ring the alarm: the crisis of black youth suicide in America. 2019. Available at: https://watsoncoleman.house.gov/uploadedfiles/full_taskforce_report.pdf.   Accessed December 20, 2021.
14. Subica AM, Wu LT. Substance use and suicide in Pacific Islander, American Indian and multiracial youth. Am J Prev Med 2018;54(6):795–805.
15. Manzo K, Hobbs GR, Gachupin FC, et al. Reservation-urban comparison of suicidal ideation/planning and attempts in American Indian youth. J Sch Health 2020;90(6):439–46.
16. Centers for Disease Control and Prevention. Web-based injury statistics query and reporting system. cdc.gov. 2020. Available at: https://www.cdc.gov/nchs/products/databriefs/db362.htm. Accessed February 6, 2021.
17. Xiao Y, Lu W. Temporal trends and disparities in suicidal behaviors by sex and sexual identity among Asian American adolescents. JAMA Netw Open 2021;4(4):e214498.
18. Hishinuma ES, Smith MD, McCarthy K, et al. Longitudinal prediction of suicide attempts for a diverse adolescent sample of Native Hawaiians, Pacific peoples, and Asian Americans. Arch Suicide Res 2018;22(1):67–90.
19. Kim JJ, Kodish T, Bear L, et al. Disparities in follow-up care for Asian American youth assessed for suicide risk in schools. Asian Am J Psychol 2018;9(4):308–17.
20. Ruch DA, Sheftall AH, Schlagbaum BS, et al. Trends in suicide among youth aged 10 to 19 years in the United States, 1975-2016. JAMA Netw Open 2019;2(5):e193886.
21. Roche KM, White RMB, Lambert SF, et al. Association of family member detention or deportation with Latino or Latina adolescents' later risks of suicidal ideation, alcohol use, and externalizing problems. JAMA Pediatr 2020;174(5):478–86.
22. Nishina A, Witkow MR. Why developmental researchers should care about biracial, multiracial, and multiethnic youth. Child Development Perspect 2019;14(1):21–7.
23. Gattamorta KA, Salerno JP, Castro AJ. Intersectionality and health behaviors among US high school students: examining race/ethnicity, sexual identity, and sex. J Sch Health 2019;89(10):800–8.
24. Baiden P, LaBrenz CA, Asiedua-Baiden G, et al. Examining the intersection of race/ethnicity and sexual orientation on suicidal ideation and suicide attempt among adolescents: findings from the 2017 your risk behavior survey. J Psychiatr Res 2020;125:13–20.
25. Feinstein BA, Turner BC, Beach LB, et al. Mental health, substance use, and bullying victimization among self-identified bisexual high school aged youth. LGBT Health 2019;6(4):174–83.
26. Meza JL, Bath E. One size does not fit all: making suicide prevention and intervention equitable for our increasingly diverse communities. J Am Acad Child Adolesc Psychiatry 2021;60(6):789.
27. Halliday-Boykins CA, Schoenwald SK, Letourneau EJ. Caregiver-therapist ethnic similarity predicts youth outcomes from an empirically based treatment. J Consult Clin Psychol 2005;73(5):808.
28. Becker KD, Boustani M, Gellatly R, et al. Forty years of engagement research in children's mental health services: multidimensional measurement and practice elements. J Clin Child Adolesc Psychol 2018;47(1):1–23.

29. Molock SD, Puri R, Matlin S, et al. Relationship between religious coping and suicidal behaviors among African American adolescents. Jour Black Psychol 2006; 32(3):366–89.

30. Goldston DB, Molock SD, Whitbeck LB, et al. Cultural considerations in adolescent suicide prevention and psychosocial treatment. Am Psychol 2008;63(1): 14–31.

31. Kim E, Kang M. The effects of client–counselor racial matching on therapeutic outcome. Asia Pac Educ Rev 2018;19:103–10.

32. Price MA, Weisz JR, McKetta S, et al. Meta-analysis: are psychotherapies less effective for black youth in communities with higher levels of anti-black racism? J Am Acad Child Adolesc Psychiatry 2021;60(8):1–10.

33. McCauley E, Berk MS, Asarnow JR, et al. Efficacy of dialectical behavior therapy for adolescents at high risk for suicide: a randomized clinical trial. JAMA Psychiatry 2018;75(8):777–85.

34. Linehan M. Special treatment strategies. Suicidal behavior strategies. Cognitive-behavioral treatment of borderline personality disorder. 1993.

35. Glenn CR, Esposito EC, Porter AC, et al. Evidence base update of psychosocial treatments for self-injurious thoughts and behaviors in youth. J Clin Child Adolesc Psychol 2019;48(3):357–92.

36. Mehlum L, Tørmoen AJ, Ramberg M, et al. Dialectical behavior therapy for adolescents with repeated suicidal and self-harming behavior: a randomized trial. J Am Acad Child Adolesc Psychiatry 2014;53(10):1082–91.

37. Mufson L, Moreau D, Weissman MM, et al. Modification of interpersonal psychotherapy with depressed adolescents (IPT-A): phase I and II studies. J Am Acad Child Adolesc Psychiatry 1994;33(5):695–705.

38. Tang T-C, Jou S-H, Ko C-H, et al. Randomized study of school-based intensive interpersonal psychotherapy for depressed adolescents with suicidal risk and parasuicide behaviors. Psychiatry Clin Neurosci 2009;63(4):463–70.

39. Frey LM, Hunt QA. Treatment for suicidal thoughts and behavior: a review of family-based interventions. J Marital Fam Ther 2018;44(1):107–24.

40. Diamond GS, Diamond GM, Levy SA. Attachment-based family therapy for depressed adolescents. 2014.

41. Diamond GS, Wintersteen MB, Brown GK, et al. Attachment-based family therapy for adolescents with suicidal ideation: a randomized controlled trial. J Am Acad Child Adolesc Psychiatry 2010;49(2):122–31.

42. Diamond GS, Kobak RR, Krauthamer Ewing ES, et al. A randomized controlled trial: attachment-based family and nondirective supportive treatments for youth who are suicidal. J Am Acad Child Adolesc Psychiatry 2019;58(7):721–31.

43. Asarnow JR, Berk M, Hughes JL, et al. The SAFETY program: a treatment-development trial of a cognitive-behavioral family treatment for adolescent suicide attempters. J Clin Child Adolesc Psychol 2015;44(1):194–203.

44. Asarnow JR, Hughes JL, Babeva KN, et al. Cognitive-behavioral family treatment for suicide attempt prevention: a randomized controlled trial. J Am Acad Child Adolesc Psychiatry 2017;56(6):506–14.

45. Ougrin D, Tranah T, Stahl D, et al. Therapeutic interventions for suicide attempts and self-harm in adolescents: systematic review and meta-analysis. J Am Acad Child Adolesc Psychiatry 2015;54(2):97–107.e2.

46. Asarnow JR, Mehlum L. Practitioner review: treatment for suicidal and self-harming adolescents – advances in suicide prevention care. J Child Psychol Psychiatry 2019;60(10):1046–54.

47. Duarte-Velez Y, Torres-Davila P, Spirito A, et al. Development of a treatment protocol for Puerto Rican adolescents with suicidal behaviors. Psychotherapy 2016; 53(1):45.
48. Robinson WL, Case MH, Whipple CR, et al. Culturally grounded stress reduction and suicide prevention for African American adolescents. Pract Innov 2016; 1(2):117.
49. Cwik M, Goklish N, Masten K, et al. Let our Apache heritage and culture live on forever and teach the young ones: development of the elders' resilience curriculum, an upstream suicide prevention approach for American Indian youth. Am J Community Psychol 2019;64(1–2):137–45.

Unpacking the Layers
Dismantling Inequities in Substance Use Services and Outcomes for Racially Minoritized Adolescents

Michelle V. Porche, EdD[a],*, Lisa R. Fortuna, MD, MPH, MDiv[b],
Marina Tolou-Shams, PhD[c]

KEYWORDS

- Substance use disorders • Access to care • Disparities
- Black, Latinx, and American Indian youth • Youth of color • Systems of care

KEY POINTS

- Racial and ethnic minority youth experience significant barriers to substance use disorder (SUD) treatment and receive lesser quality services than their White counterparts in the United States.
- Black and Latinx adolescents are less likely than White adolescents to receive treatment of SUDs or to have close geographic proximity to SUD treatment facilities.
- Inequities in access to care result in significant disparate outcomes for Black, Latinx, and American Indian youth including disrupted education, juvenile detention, economic disparities, and poor mental health.
- Integration of services in primary care and schools could offer expanded access to prevention and treatment, especially for cannabis use and mild to moderate disorders.
- Collaboration among community health and mental health centers should improve access to culturally and structurally responsive care for patients in geographic areas with limited health care resources.

Note: The first two authors contributed equally.
[a] Department of Psychiatry and Behavioral Sciences, Zuckerberg San Francisco General Hospital and Trauma Center, University of California, San Francisco (UCSF), 1001 Potrero Avenue, Building 5, Room 7M, San Francisco, CA, USA; [b] Department of Psychiatry and Behavioral Sciences, Zuckerberg San Francisco General Hospital and Trauma Center, University of California, San Francisco, 1001 Potrero Avenue, Building 5, Room 7M16, San Francisco, CA, USA; [c] Department of Psychiatry and Behavioral Sciences, Zuckerberg San Francisco General Hospital and Trauma Center, University of California, San Francisco, 1001 Potrero Avenue, Building 5, Room 7M18, San Francisco, CA 94110, USA
* Corresponding author.
E-mail address: michelle.porche@ucsf.edu
Twitter: @michellevporche (M.V.P.)

Child Adolesc Psychiatric Clin N Am 31 (2022) 223–236
https://doi.org/10.1016/j.chc.2021.11.002
1056-4993/22/© 2021 Elsevier Inc. All rights reserved.

childpsych.theclinics.com

BACKGROUND

Substance use problems remain a significant public health concern for minoritized youth. Our review emphasizes the urgency of addressing service gaps, given that youth of color who have substance use disorders (SUD) and mental health disorders before age 18 have worse education, employment, and social outcomes than those with later onset or no SUD[1,2] Although youth of color are not more likely to suffer a SUD, as compared with their White counterparts, those that do are less likely to receive treatment services in the community, and more likely to be involved in the justice and/or child welfare system. In this article, we review the existing literature on substance use services for adolescents and discuss implications for disparate outcomes by race, ethnicity, and gender. We reflect on the complex, intersectional layers of inequities, and recommend ways that child-serving systems can work toward improving SUD services for Black, Latinx, American Indian, and other youth of color. We describe data from the National Survey on Drug Use and Health (NSUDH) along with findings from other substance use treatment trials conducted with specific groups of minoritized youth, such as girls involved in the juvenile justice system. The NSUDH data provide the estimates of substance use and mental illness at the national, state, and substate levels. Substance use intervention trials with justice-involved girls provide insight into a particularly underserved population given that they represent a smaller subpopulation of youth in the justice system and services need to be designed for their specific needs, including intersectional identities as young women who are disproportionately Black, Latinx, and American Indian/Native Alaskan. The topic of efficacious substance use interventions for young people of color is overwhelmingly underaddressed in clinical services and research. A review of controlled treatment studies found that few studies intentionally considered differences in outcomes by race or ethnicity in their design and fewer conducted statistical tests of difference.[3]

Finally, the authors share promising approaches to improving prevention and treatment options for problematic substance use, including practical strategies for improving access and addressing social, structural, and cultural barriers to SUD services for the youth of color.

Social Determinants, Policies, and Substance Use Disorder Disparities

There are several social determinants, which influence the course of SUD and with differential consequences for Black, Latinx, and other youth of color. The social and physical environments play an important role, in particular, to the risk for the development of SUD and appropriate access and quality of care for SUD in minoritized youth. For example, alcohol outlet (sales) density remains far greater in Black and Hispanic/Latinx neighborhoods than for majority White neighborhoods.[4] Social economic factors, including poverty, are important contributors to services disparities, as are cultural and structural barriers. Research shows that Black and American Indian clients are less likely to initiate or engage in treatment compared with non-Latino White clients.[5] American Indian clients living in economically disadvantaged communities are at even greater risk of not initiating treatment than their counterparts living in better-resourced communities.[6] The combination of these findings suggest that there is a lack of accessible, culturally appropriate substance use services for youth residing in primary communities of color.[7]

The epidemiologic data demonstrate differences in SUD services, need, use, and access by race and gender. Data from National Survey on Drug Use and Health, 2019 release, show that White youth have double the rate of outpatient treatment initiation as compared with Black youth (**Table 1**). Often entering into substance use

Table 1
Prevalence of past-year abuse or dependence and treatment by race national survey on drug use and health, 2019 cohort

	Non-Latino White % (SE)	Latino % (SE)	Asian % (SE)	Black % (SE)	Native American % (SE)
Participants with substance abuse or dependence in previous year	4.76% (0.35%)	5.47% (0.66%)	1.20% (0.59%)	3.93% (0.57%)	9.06% (2.58%)
Specialty treatment past 12 mo	0.34% (0.09)	0.19% (0.11%)	N/A	0.40% (0.15%)	N/A
Informal treatment past 12 mo	0.67% (0.12%)	1.08% (0.29%)	0.10% (0.10%)	0.64% (0.22%)	2.35% (1.40%)
Emotional treatment in jail or juvenile detention past 12 mo	0.10% (0.04%)	0.09% (0.05%)	N/A	0.90% (0.30%)	0.74% (0.74%)

Substance Abuse and Mental Health Services Administration. (2020). Key substance use and mental health indicators in the United States: Results from the 2019 National Survey on Drug Use and Health (HHS Publication No. PEP20-07-01-001, NSDUH Series H-55). Rockville, MD: Center for Behavioral Health Statistics and Quality, Substance Abuse and Mental Health Services Administration. Retrieved from https://www.samhsa.gov/data/.

treatment with greater severity of SUD symptoms and/or related consequences, youth of color experience more barriers to treatment engagement, completion, and are less satisfied with the care they receive than their White counterparts are.[8,9] Compared with non-Latino Whites with SUD, Black, and Latinx adolescents with SUD report receiving lesser quality and intensity of care.[5] In regard to overall access, White youth receive double the rate of outpatient treatment compared with Black youth. In a study of 664 youth receiving intensive case management, those with substance use were less likely to come from racial/ethnic minority groups.[10]

The lack of focus on evidence-based SUD prevention research in minoritized communities and lack of access to secondary prevention interventions such as overdose education and naltrexone distribution programs by the youth of color further contribute to disparities.[11] This includes: the lower availability of evidence-based treatment (particularly buprenorphine), the unequal deployment of drug testing with markedly different consequences for minoritized youth when their test results are positive (ie, juvenile justice vs treatment; increased likelihood of being pushed out of the school system), and, markedly different rates of juvenile detention despite national survey data that suggest that minoritized youth use drugs at similar rates as White youth.

INTERSECTIONALITY OF RACE AND GENDER AND POPULATIONS WITHIN SETTINGS SUCH AS SCHOOLS

An early systematic review of 46 studies found consistent associations between elevated use of substances and high school dropout, although the indicators for increased risk for Black and Latino youth were mixed.[12] Further research has investigated predictors of substance use as well as its explanatory power for understanding school outcomes. Childhood trauma was identified as a precursor to both conduct disorder and substance use, which acted as mediators of high school dropout for a national community sample; rates were highest for Latino youth, above the national average for Black youth, and lowest for Asian youth except for Southeast Asians that dropped out at similar rates to Latino students.[13] These results are illustrative of the heterogeneity of racial and ethnic categories. Importantly, 38% of this sample reported one or more major trauma experience, and 32% were identified as having one or more DSM-IV diagnosis (in use at the time of the study).[13] However, only 17% reported receiving any mental health services as a child. Data from youth in the Longitudinal Studies of Child Use and Neglect, which was comprised primarily of minoritized youth (54% Black, 6% Latino, 14% mixed race or other race), found direct links between the number of ACEs and dropout, and specifically that having a household member with substance use, as well as individual externalizing problems and peers that used substances, were also identified as risk factors for dropout.[14] These studies point to the need for school-based services that can address trauma and support or provide mental health treatment, while decreasing reliance on harsh punishment in response to substance use and externalizing symptoms.

With the pandemic came patterns of increased alcohol and cannabis use which was not only problematic for youth using substances in isolation but also increased risk for COVID-19 transmission when using with peers.[15] Schools, of which the majority were operating remotely during the pandemic, serve as important sites of social connection with peers, including increasing emphasis on the digital connection of texting.[16] Close relationships with parents and prosocial peers are protective for substance use, though increased risk for youth is associated with peers who engage in delinquency behaviors.[17] To better understand the sequence of use patterns, progression of risk behaviors and academic outcomes was illuminated through longitudinal analysis of the Add Health study that found that failing courses predicted later alcohol use, whereas alcohol use did not predict increased failure of coursework.[18]

Extracurricular activities have been found to be protective against adolescent substance use generally.[19] Research on American Indian adolescents found that higher perceived availability of activities and higher frequency and intensity of involvement were associated with lower rates of substance use[20] indicating the importance of extracurricular opportunities in school settings and communities as prevention policy. Conversely, research about decision-making regarding drug use underscores the role of context for youth in determining which settings are more conducive to substance use.[21] A multi-level analysis including 34 schools in the mid-west found that students in schools with clear norms discouraging use and with higher proportions of Black and Latinx peers were less likely to use substances; these school setting characteristics also moderated the influence of substance-using peers.[22]

Investigation of adolescent perception of drugs as harmful or helpful is critical for prevention and intervention development. A study of sexual and gender individuals assigned female at birth found higher levels of alcohol and cannabis use correlated with minority stressors and higher rates of anxiety and depression symptoms.[23] A retrospective study of Puerto Rican prison inmates found a significant association between childhood symptoms of ADHD (though not necessarily a formal diagnosis) and lifetime and current SUD (often leading to sentencing), and comorbid anxiety, depression, or PTSD.[24] Analysis of historical trends for the Monitoring the Future Study from 1976 to 2019 found increasing rates of lifetime cannabis use for boys than girls and Black adolescents than other racial groups.[25] There is some speculation as to whether these increases are related to policy changes in legalization. Further research with adolescents would illuminate the onset of these beliefs and patterns.

ILLUSTRATIVE VIGNETTE

We present a vignette based on a mixed-methods study of youth in an acute specialty care detoxification facility,[26] to show complex and multiple individual and structural risk factors for a 17-year-old Black girl in treatment of cannabis and tobacco dependency. By the time this adolescent girl entered a treatment facility she had been through eight foster care placements and multiple times in juvenile detention for "pot and behavior" and was at the time on probation for receiving stolen property. Black and Latinx families are disproportionately represented in Family and Children's Services, and the family itself is less likely to receive support necessary to keep children from being separated from parents, often placing children on a detrimental path through the foster care system. These dual-status youth experience persistent complex trauma and systemic trauma while moving through child welfare and the justice system.[27] This is a teenager with little family support, racially isolated at a predominantly White school, and with few positive connections to adults. She describes some support from school, "they don't know what's going on... My French teacher [and the] class wrote a letter for me in French. It's a small school, like 500 kids and I'm one of four Black girls." Despite this positive attention and connection with her French teacher, no one notices that her drug use is affecting her academic engagement and achievement, "I always used to get high before school so... I'd be tired by like 4th period though, I'd be just wanting to go to sleep, lie down, smoke again." Failed by multiple systems, she will likely age out of foster care with the continued need of trauma-focused treatment of addiction.

Gender socialization and social learning can influence risk behaviors, including the initiation and patterns of drug and alcohol use.[28–31] Specifically, research by Akers[32] on substance use focuses on the aspects of social learning that influence gender differences: including modeling (imitation), differential reinforcement (balance of reward and punishment), and definitions (balance of attitudes favorable and unfavorable toward the behavior). There is a need for more research highlighting the importance of, and more closely examining, racial–ethnic differences in justice populations. There are likely to be differing health needs, and subsequent treatment approaches, by racial/ethnic group and by gender.

JUSTICE INVOLVED YOUTH

Despite overall declines in youth arrest rates since 2010, estimates indicate approximately 697,000 youth under the age of 18 are arrested annually.[33] Rates of decline, however, are substantially lower for women (31% of 2019 arrests) and rates of disproportionate arrest for Black youth persist. American Indian youth also have disproportionate arrest rates relative to White youth but rates among Latinx youth are not uniformly reported and therefore unknown.[33] Juvenile justice system contact is associated with a variety of adverse public health outcomes, such as substance use,[34–36] psychiatric symptoms,[36–38] sexual risk behavior,[34,39] and higher rates of sexually transmitted infections (STIs).[40–42] As many as 50% of justice-involved youth who use substances also have ADHD; rates of traumatic violence exposure are astronomically high and associated with symptoms of posttraumatic stress and increased rates of problematic substance use. Much of prior research focuses on these associations among youth in detention; more recent research demonstrates these same adverse public health outcomes hold for youth who may have had only one court contact, even if never detained (herein referred to as justice-impacted youth or JIY).[34,43,44] For example, first-time justice-involved youth who are on average 14.5 years old report 3 prior adverse childhood experiences (ACEs) and those ACEs, particularly abuse, are associated with problematic substance use and mental health needs 1 year later.

Additionally, substance use is associated with recidivism for youth and adults with co-occurring mental health needs.[36,45,46] Teplin and colleagues[47] have conducted seminal work on the long-term (up to 15 years) trajectories of substance use and psychiatric disorders in a juvenile detainee sample demonstrating high rates of psychiatric and comorbid substance use need that follows a diverse cohort of JIY into young adulthood.[47] The US juvenile justice system has largely become the default behavioral health system of care and primary setting for SUD treatment of minoritized youth, which only serves to perpetuate systems of racial oppression and mass incarceration that are responsible in the first place for the gross inequities in community-based substance use services access and associated poorer health outcomes for minoritized youth into adulthood.

Promising Culturally Responsive Interventions and Evidence-Based Treatment

Systematic analysis of primary substance use prevention programs for children and adolescents[48] described a final pool of 90 studies on 16 different programs, but of that group most reported on majority White or nonidentified samples. Only 4 included specificity for a Black sample, 3 for a Latinx sample, and two with an American Indian sample, suggesting limited attention to cultural factors in prevention design. Meta-analysis[7] identified 8 peer-reviewed publications describing culturally sensitive programs out of more than 7000 searched. These culturally sensitive treatments were specifically designed for Black, Hispanic, or Native American youth. Some included multi-lingual delivery, cultural competency training of clinicians, racial-ethnic matching of provider to client, and offering accessible locations. These adapted interventions showed a significantly larger reduction in symptoms relative to comparison conditions.

Attrition is a significant problem in working with adolescents in general and even more so among adolescents with substance use problems. Fortuna, Porche, and Padilla[49] conducted an open pilot trial study of a manualized therapy for adolescents with posttraumatic stress, depression, and substance use that uses a combination of cognitive therapy and mindfulness, and delivered in the preferred language of the youth (English or Spanish) in community-based settings (eg, primary care, community-based organizations and community mental health clinics). The study had a 62% retention rate, not dissimilar to other treatment studies with adolescents for depression, anxiety, PTSD, and SUDs. Latinx adolescents had a higher rate of retention than other participants did; the opportunity to work with a culturally matched Spanish-speaking provider may have been an influence. In addition, the therapy intervention was developed with input from youth, including Latinx immigrants, to better understand relevant terminology, and socio-cultural context of their trauma experiences. The significance of integrating spirituality was an important theme. Overall, youth outcomes provided evidence of decreased substance use and reduced PTSD symptoms.[49]

FAMILY-BASED INTERVENTIONS

Research demonstrates that treatment, recovery, and family well-being outcomes improve when the complex needs of each family member are met through supportive services. The Multiple-Family Group Intervention (MFGI) was developed for use with boys and girls from diverse backgrounds in juvenile justice.[50] To address affect regulation and attachment, youth and families participated in an 8-week session of family therapy that used video, discussion, and roleplay, before release from juvenile correctional facilities. Results at 6-month follow-up showed improved caregiver-child relationships, reduced attachment to delinquent peers, reduction in recidivism, decline in externalizing behaviors, and significant reduction in drug and alcohol use.[50] One of the few available interventions working with Spanish-speaking Latinx immigrant parents provided an 8-week intervention to improve parenting practices associated with risk of adolescent substance use including harsh parenting, monitoring, conflict, attachment, and involvement.[51] Designed in collaboration with Latinx parents and community groups, the intervention showed evidence of feasibility and of improving parent–child relationships that would be protective against adolescent substance use.[51] A family-centered approach extends well beyond the SUD treatment system and includes the child welfare system, courts, and mental health services, and includes all other agencies and individuals who interact with and serve families.

Gender-Based Intervention, with Girls of Color

Recent cannabis use rates among 14.5-year-old (8–10th graders) justice-involved youth living in the community are approximately 50%[34]; this is more than twice that reported by 12th graders in general adolescent population surveys.[52] Justice-involved youth report higher rates of cannabis use (48% of community-supervised; 54% of detained youth) than their same-age non-justice-involved peers, and often begin using cannabis by 13 year old.[34,53] Youth arrested in the past year have over 6 times higher prevalence of cannabis use disorder compared with those with no past year justice involvement.[54] Rates of cannabis use are particularly high among justice-involved girls in the community, with 55% reporting lifetime use (vs 45% of boys).[34] Cannabis use has significant consequences for justice-involved youth, with those who report past year use being more likely to experience school failure, use other substances, sell and be offered drugs, and engage in violent behavior.[55] Despite being highly prevalent with these far-ranging consequences, community supervised justice-involved youth are unlikely to receive substance use services; only 33% of community supervision and behavioral health providers serving justice-involved youth provide such services.[56] Motivational enhancement therapy/cognitive behavioral therapy (MET/CBT) is a widely used, evidence-based adolescent group-based substance use intervention, including for justice-involved youth.[57] Yet, of the 600 Cannabis Youth Trial (CYT) participants (including 62% justice-involved),[58] most were men (83%) and White (61%).[59,60] A recent MI/CBT trial included 65% racial and ethnic minority incarcerated youth but only 10% girls and MI/CBT was not superior to relaxation training and substance education/12 steps in reducing youth cannabis use.[61] Despite widespread dissemination, we lack studies of MET/CBT efficacy or effectiveness in reducing cannabis use with larger samples of justice-involved girls and/or Black and Latinx youth.

Data suggest girls have unique developmental pathways to substance use and justice system involvement, warranting *gender-responsive* intervention. Justice-involved girls experience substantially higher rates of trauma, abuse (all types), and neglect than boys, which is associated with girls' increased substance use and more severe psychopathology (particularly internalizing disorders such as depression). These worse behavioral health outcomes are also correlated with juvenile justice involvement.[62,63] Likewise, conflictual interpersonal relationships seem to be related to girls' substance use, sexual and reproductive health, and delinquency.[64–66] Certain psychological constructs, such as self-efficacy, self-esteem, empowerment, and identity (eg, related to gender, race, and ethnicity) are also related to girls' health and behavioral outcomes[67–69] including cannabis use patterns.[70] Gender-responsive substance use interventions targeting these constructs and addressing unique developmental pathways to risk (eg, are trauma-informed), such as Helping Women Recover, reduce substance use and recidivism[71,72] among women in the criminal justice system.

VOICES is the adolescent version of Helping Women Recover[73] and the first gender-responsive trauma-informed substance use intervention developed specifically for justice-involved girls. VOICES includes content corresponding with Markoff and colleagues's[74] 10 principles of trauma-informed care,[74] such as emphasizing strengths and resilience and recognizing the impact of violence and victimization on development and coping strategies. All activities are based on relational and gender empowerment theories. Drug use, mental health, and well-being are addressed in intervention activities promoting learning and understanding of feelings about self and interpersonal relationships. Unlike CBT approaches that directly target substance use attitudes, beliefs, feelings, and behaviors and teach coping, refusal, and emotion regulation skills to reduce use,[75] VOICES aims to build girls' empowerment, resiliency, and positive relationships to protect girls from future substance use. A recently published trial of the VOICES intervention with 113 justice and school-referred girls, ages 12 to 17 years old, with a lifetime history of substance use demonstrated that rates of cannabis use at 9-month postbaseline were significantly lower for girls randomized to VOICES 12 session, 1-hour weekly group intervention compared with a psychoeducational didactic control group (GirlHealth) matched for time and attention.[76] Cannabis use decreased from 56% at baseline to 38% at month 9 in the VOICES group, while use in the GH group increased from 51% to 61%. The interaction between the type and duration of time of the intervention was statistically significant ($F = 2.92$, $P = .03$). Similar differences were observed in biologically (urine toxicology) confirmed cannabis use; cannabis was detected in 28% of the VOICES group at baseline and 19% at month 9%, and 27% of the GH group at baseline and 39% at month 9 (intervention x time, $F = 2.28$, $P = .08$). Statistically significant decreases in trauma and depression symptoms, as well as cannabis- and alcohol-related consequences, were observed in both groups, potentially reflecting a general benefit of group intervention. Delivery of VOICES by telehealth and new research in this area have created a new opportunity for reaching girls.

SUMMARY

Black, Latinx, Native American, and other youth of color are less likely than White adolescents to receive treatment of SUDs, the vast majority of which involve marijuana and alcohol misuse. Minority youth are less likely to have health insurance, to be identified and referred for SUD, and to have close geographic proximity to SUD treatment facilities. A multitude of economic, social, environmental, gender, cultural, and individual factors contribute to access gaps. Inequities in access to care result in consequentially disparate outcomes for minoritized youth including disrupted education, incarceration, economic disparities, and poor mental health.

Preventative and interventional services integration in primary care and schools could offer expanded access to treatment, and collaboration with the community could improve access to culturally and structurally responsive care for patients in geographic areas with limited health care resources. Adolescents who do not address their alcohol and drug use can experience lifelong mental health and economic consequences. Child and Adolescent Providers and policymakers must advocate for expanded coverage and access to SUD prevention and treatment, implementation, reimbursed, and integrated SUD and mental health services that are culturally appropriate, equitable, and antiracist, and trauma informed within child-serving systems of care.

PRACTICAL RECOMMENDATIONS

Policy

1. Advocate for policies aimed at expanding coverage and access to SUD prevention and treatment that is local and accessible for communities of color.
2. Adopt state policies and regulations that increase eligibility and coverage of basic substance-use treatments for youth with public insurance.
3. Leverage juvenile justice reform to promote concurrent policy changes in adolescent SUD prevention, identification, and treatment access.

Services

4. Integrate SUD and mental health services, which are culturally appropriate, equitable, antiracist, and trauma-informed across child-serving systems of care.
5. Improve access to culturally, structurally competent, and gender appropriate care for patients in geographic areas with limited health care resources.
6. Intervene at multiple, critical points of justice system contact to improve youth behavioral health, legal, and other associated outcomes.
7. Develop school-based messaging about substance use norms that are based on building connections with students, and approach prevention and intervention through a trauma-sensitive lens, including attention to racial trauma; encourage self-reflection for staff regarding racial bias and expectations.
8. Advance public health initiatives, which promote and incentivize assessment, identification, and referral of SUDs across child and family-serving systems.

RESEARCH

1. Include minoritized youth and girls in study designs.
2. Develop culturally specific and intergenerational interventions (eg, development and testing of holistic substance use interventions that treat substance using caregiver and youth within a family-based intervention).
3. Research services innovations and their implementation across child-serving systems (eg, studying interorganizational relationships and cross-system collaborative strategies that successfully expand care access).
4. Implement learning collaboratives to increase access and capacity for substance use treatment in community-based services.
5. Create and test digital health interventions for SUD prevention and treatment and study outcomes for minoritized youth (eg, hybrid design trials of SUD group treatment of special populations, like girls, delivered via telehealth).

CLINICS CARE POINTS

- Implement universal screening with substance use screening tools, such as the CRAFFT, to identify adolescents at risk, and in need of further assessment of substance disorders in primary care and mental health services.

- Conduct a comprehensive diagnostic evaluation that includes the youth and their caregivers to characterize developmental history, risk, and protective factors, history of trauma and adversity, current and lifetime psychiatric symptoms and disorders, and substance use and related disorders.

- Use of the updated cultural formulation model is strongly advised at intake with youth of color to understand their causal attributions, cultural conceptions of coping, and help seeking for substance use.

- All adolescents who present with substance use or SUDs need to be carefully assessed for co-occurring psychiatric disorders.

- Use of culturally responsive and trauma informed evidence-based behavioral interventions should be used as the foundation or platform for treating adolescents with SUDs and whenever possible, include their families in treatment.

- Prescription of pharmacologic treatment should be administered appropriately for non-SUD disorders and without bias. For example, youth diagnosed with ADHD should not be denied stimulant medications designed to address this neurodevelopmental condition, even while receiving treatment for SUD.

DISCLOSURE

Writing support for the first and third authors was provided by the California Institute on Law, Neuroscience, and Education at UCSF.

REFERENCES

1. Brook JS, Adams RE, Balka EB, et al. Early adolescent marijuana use: risks for the transition to young adulthood. Psychol Med 2002;32(1):79–91.
2. Brown TL, Flory K, Lynam DR, et al. Comparing the developmental trajectories of marijuana use of African American and Caucasian adolescents: patterns, antecedents, and consequences. Exp Clin Psychopharmacol 2004;12(1): 47–56.
3. Strada MJ, Donohue B, Lefforge NL. Examination of ethnicity in controlled treatment outcome studies involving adolescent substance abusers: a comprehensive literature review. Psychol Addict Behav 2006;20(1):11–27.
4. Romley JA, Cohen D, Ringel J, et al. Alcohol and environmental justice: the density of liquor stores and bars in urban neighborhoods in the United States. J Stud Alcohol Drugs 2007;68(1):48–55.
5. Alegria M, Carson NJ, Goncalves M, et al. Disparities in treatment for substance use disorders and co-occurring disorders for ethnic/racial minority youth. J Am Acad Child Adolesc Psychiatry 2011;50(1):22–31.
6. Campbell CI, Weisner C, Sterling S. Adolescents entering chemical dependency treatment in private managed care: ethnic differences in treatment initiation and retention. J Adolesc Health 2006;38(4):343–50.
7. Steinka-Fry KT, Tanner-Smith EE, Dakof GA, et al. Culturally sensitive substance use treatment for racial/ethnic minority youth: a meta-analytic review. J Subst Abuse Treat 2017;75:22–37.
8. Linton SL, Winiker A, Tormohlen KN, et al. "People Don't Just Start Shooting Heroin on Their 18th Birthday": a qualitative study of community stakeholders' perspectives on adolescent opioid use and opportunities for intervention in Baltimore, Maryland. Prev Sci 2021;22(5):621–32.
9. Wu L-T, Blazer DG, Li T-K, et al. Treatment use and barriers among adolescents with prescription opioid use disorders. Addict Behav 2011;36(12):1233–9.
10. Evans ME, Dollard N, McNulty TL. Characteristics of seriously emotionally disturbed youth with and without substance abuse in intensive case management. J Child Fam Stud 1992;1(3):305–14.
11. Hadland SE, Wharam JF, Schuster MA, et al. Trends in receipt of buprenorphine and naltrexone for opioid use disorder among adolescents and young adults, 2001-2014. JAMA Pediatr 2017;171(8):747.

12. Townsend L, Flisher AJ, King G. A systematic review of the relationship between high school dropout and substance use. Clin Child Fam Psychol Rev 2007;10(4): 295–317.

13. Porche MV, Fortuna LR, Lin J, et al. Childhood trauma and psychiatric disorders as correlates of school dropout in a national sample of young adults. Child Dev 2011;82(3):982–98.

14. Morrow AS, Villodas MT. Direct and indirect pathways from adverse childhood experiences to high school dropout among high-risk adolescents. J Res Adolesc 2018;28(2):327–41.

15. Dumas TM, Ellis W, Litt DM. What does adolescent substance use look like during the COVID-19 pandemic? Examining changes in frequency, social contexts, and pandemic-related predictors. J Adolesc Health 2020;67(3):354–61.

16. Tulane S, Vaterlaus JM, Beckert TE. An A in their social lives, but an F in school: adolescent perceptions of texting in school. Youth Soc 2017;49(6):711–32.

17. Lombardi CM, Coley RL, Sims J, et al. Social norms, social connections, and sex differences in adolescent mental and behavioral health. J Child Fam Stud 2019; 28(1):91–104.

18. Crosnoe R. The connection between academic failure and adolescent drinking in secondary school. Sociol Educ 2006;79(1):44–60.

19. Elder C. Organized group activity as a protective factor against adolescent substance use. Am J Health Behav 2000;24(2). https://doi.org/10.5993/AJHB.24.2.3.

20. Moilanen KL, Markstrom CA, Jones E. Extracurricular activity availability and participation and substance use among American Indian adolescents. J Youth Adolesc 2014;43(3):454–69.

21. Price Wolf J, Lipperman-Kreda S, Bersamin M. "It just Depends on the Environment": patterns and decisions of substance use and co-use by adolescents. J Child Adolesc Subst Abuse 2019;28(3):143–9.

22. Su J, Supple AJ. School substance use norms and racial composition moderate parental and peer influences on adolescent substance use. Am J Community Psychol 2016;57(3–4):280–90.

23. Dyar C, Sarno EL, Newcomb ME, et al. Longitudinal associations between minority stress, internalizing symptoms, and substance use among sexual and gender minority individuals assigned female at birth. J Consulting Clin Psychol 2020; 88(5):389–401.

24. González RA, Vélez-Pastrana MC, Ruiz Varcárcel JJ, et al. Childhood ADHD symptoms are associated with lifetime and current illicit substance-use disorders and in-site health risk behaviors in a representative sample of Latino prison inmates. J Atten Disord 2015;19(4):301–12.

25. Terry-McElrath YM, O'Malley PM, Johnston LD. The growing transition from lifetime marijuana use to frequent use among 12th grade students: U.S. National data from 1976 to 2019. Drug Alcohol Depend 2020;212:108064.

26. Fortuna LR, Porche MV, Alam N, et al. Smoking and co-occurring disorders: implications for smoking Cessation interventions for adolescents in residential addiction treatment. J Dual Diagn 2012;8(2):133–9.

27. Simmons-Horton SY. "A Bad combination": Lived experiences of youth involved in the foster care and juvenile justice systems. Child Adolesc Soc Work J 2020. https://doi.org/10.1007/s10560-020-00693-1.

28. Akers RL, Lee G. Age, social learning, and social bonding in adolescent substance use. Deviant Behav 1999;20(1):1–25.

29. Mahalik JR, Burns SM, Syzdek M. Masculinity and perceived normative health behaviors as predictors of men's health behaviors. Soc Sci Med 2007;64(11): 2201–9.
30. Raffaelli M, Torres Stone RA, Iturbide MI, et al. Acculturation, gender, and alcohol use among Mexican American college students. Addict Behav 2007;32(10): 2187–99.
31. White HR, Jackson K. Social and psychological influences on emerging adult drinking behavior. Alcohol Res Health 2004;28(4):182–90.
32. Akers RL. Social learning and social structure: a general theory of crime and deviance, 2009, New York: Routledge.
33. Puzzanchera C. Juvenile arrests, 2019. Published online 2021:16. Available at: https://ojjdp.ojp.gov/publications/juvenile-arrests-2019.pdf. Accessed December 13, 2021.
34. Tolou-Shams M, Brown LK, Marshall BDL, et al. The behavioral health needs of first-time offending justice-involved youth: substance use, sexual risk, and mental health. J Child Adolesc Subst Abuse 2019;28(5):291–303.
35. Dembo R, Jainchill N, Turner C, et al. Levels of psychopathy and its correlates: a study of incarcerated youths in three states. Behav Sci L 2007;25(5):717–38.
36. Tolou-Shams M, Rizzo CJ, Conrad SM, et al. Predictors of detention among juveniles referred for a court clinic forensic evaluation. J Am Acad Psychiatry L 2014; 42(1):56–65.
37. Abram KM, Teplin LA, McClelland GM, et al. Comorbid psychiatric disorders in youth in juvenile detention. Arch Gen Psychiatry 2003;60(11):1097–108.
38. Teplin LA, Abram KM, McClelland GM, et al. Psychiatric disorders in youth in juvenile detention. Arch Gen Psychiatry 2002;59(12):1133–43.
39. Elkington KS, Teplin LA, Mericle AA, et al. HIV/Sexually transmitted infection risk behaviors in delinquent youth with psychiatric disorders: a longitudinal study. J Am Acad Child Adolesc Psychiatry 2008;47(8):901–11.
40. Belenko S, Dembo R, Weiland D, et al. Recently arrested adolescents are at high risk for sexually transmitted diseases. Sex Transm Dis 2008;35(8):758–63.
41. Dembo R, Belenko S, Childs K, et al. Gender differences in drug use, sexually transmitted diseases, and risky sexual behavior among arrested youths. J Child Adolesc Subst Abuse 2010;19(5):424–46.
42. Tolou-Shams M, Harrison A, Hirschtritt ME, et al. Substance use and HIV among justice-involved youth: intersecting risks. Curr HIV/AIDS Rep 2019;16(1):37–47.
43. Rosen B, Dauria E, Shumway M, et al. Pregnancy attitudes, intentions and related risks among court-involved non-incarcerated youth. Published online Under review.
44. Hirschtritt ME, Dauria ED, Marshall, et al. Sexual minority, justice-involved youth: a hidden population in need of integrated mental health, substance use, and sexual health services. J Adolesc Health 2018;63:421–8.
45. Tolou-Shams M, Folk JB, Holloway ED, et al. Psychiatric and substance related problems predict recidivism for first-time justice-involved youth. Published online Under review.
46. Zgoba KM, Reeves R, Tamburello A, et al. Criminal recidivism in inmates with mental illness and substance use disorders. J Am Acad Psychiatry L 2020; 48(2):7.
47. Teplin LA, Potthoff LM, Aaby DA, et al. Prevalence, comorbidity, and continuity of psychiatric disorders in a 15-year longitudinal study of youths involved in the juvenile justice system. JAMA Pediatr 2021;175(7):e205807.

48. Tremblay M, Baydala L, Khan M, et al. Primary substance use prevention programs for children and youth: a systematic review. Pediatrics 2020;146(3): e20192747.
49. Fortuna LR, Porche MV, Padilla A. A treatment development study of a cognitive and mindfulness-based therapy for adolescents with co-occurring post-traumatic stress and substance use disorder. Psychol Psychother Theor Res Pract 2018; 91(1):42–62.
50. Keiley MK. Multiple-family group intervention for incarcerated adolescents and their families: a pilot project. J Marital Fam Ther 2007;33(1):106–24.
51. Allen ML, Hurtado GA, Yon KJ, et al. Feasibility of a parenting program to prevent substance use among Latino youth: a community-based participatory research study. Am J Health Promot 2013;27(4):240–4.
52. National Institute on Drug Abuse. Monitoring the future survey: high school and youth trends drug Facts. 2019. https://www.drugabuse.gov/publications/drugfacts/monitoring-future-survey-high-school-youth-trends. Accessed August 6, 2020.
53. Grigorenko EL, Edwards L, Chapman J. Cannabis use among juvenile detainees: typology, frequency and association. Crim Behav Ment Health 2015;25(1):54–65.
54. Winkelman TNA, Frank JW, Binswanger IA, et al. Health conditions and racial differences among justice-involved adolescents, 2009 to 2014. Acad Pediatr 2017; 17(7):723–31.
55. Vaughn MG, AbiNader M, Salas-Wright CP, et al. Trends in cannabis use among justice-involved youth in the United States, 2002–2017. Am J Drug Alcohol Abuse 2020;46(4):462–71.
56. Funk R, Knudsen HK, McReynolds LS, et al. Substance use prevention services in juvenile justice and behavioral health: results from a national survey. Health Justice 2020;8(1):1–8.
57. National Council of Juvenile and Family Court Judges. Adolescent-based treatment interventions and assessment Instruments. Available at: https://www.ncjfcj.org/wp-content/uploads/2020/04/Final-Treatment-Database-Pages.pdf. Accessed December 13, 2021.
58. Webb CPM, Burleson JA, Ungemack JA. Treating juvenile offenders for marijuana problems. Addiction 2002;97(s1):35–45.
59. Dennis M, Godley SH, Diamond G, et al. The cannabis youth treatment (CYT) study: main findings from two randomized trials. J Subst Abuse Treat 2004; 27(3):197–213.
60. Dennis M, Titus J, Diamond G, et al. The cannabis youth treatment (CYT) experiment: rationale, study design and analysis plans - Dennis - 2002 - addiction - Wiley online Library. Spec Issue Treat Marijuana Disord 2002;97(11):16–34.
61. Stein LAR, Martin R, Clair-Michaud M, et al. A randomized clinical trial of motivational interviewing plus skills training vs. relaxation plus education and 12-Steps for substance using incarcerated youth: Effects on alcohol, marijuana and crimes of aggression. Drug Alcohol Depend 2020;207:107774.
62. Abram KM, Washburn JJ, Teplin LA, et al. Posttraumatic stress disorder and psychiatric comorbidity among detained youths. Psychiatr Serv 2007;58(10):1311–6.
63. Teplin LA, Mericle AA, McClelland GM, et al. HIV and AIDS risk behaviors in juvenile detainees: implications for public health policy. Am J Public Health 2003; 93(6):906–12.
64. Owen B. In the mix: struggle and survival in a women's prison, 1998, New York: SUNY Press.66. In: Chesney-Lind M, Pasko L, editors. The female offender: girls, women, and crime, 2013, Thousand Oaks: SAGE Publications.

65. Owen B, Bloom B. Profiling women prisoners: findings from national surveys and a California sample. Prison J 1995;75(2):165–85.

66. Chesney-Lind M, Pasko L. The female offender: girls, women, and crime. SAGE Publications; 2012.

67. De La Rosa M, Dillon FR, Rojas P, et al. Latina Mother–Daughter Dyads: Relations between attachment and sexual behavior under the influence of alcohol or drugs. Arch Sex Behav 2010;39(6):1305–19.

68. Guthrie B, Flinchbaugh L. Gender-specific substance prevention programming: going beyond just focusing on girls. J Early Adolesc 2001;21(3):354–72.

69. Khoury EL. Are girls different? A developmental perspective on gender differences in risk factors for substance use among adolescents, In: Vega WA, Gil AG, editors. Drug use and ethnicity in early adolescence. Longitudinal research in the social and behavioral Sciences: an Interdisciplinary Series, 2002, New York: Kluwer, 95–123.

70. Hemsing N, Greaves L. Gender norms, roles and relations and cannabis-use patterns: a scoping review. Int J Environ Res Public Health 2020;17(3):947.

71. Messina N, Grella CE, Cartier J, et al. A randomized experimental study of gender-responsive substance abuse treatment for women in prison. J Subst Abuse Treat 2010;38(2):97–107.

72. Prendergast ML, Messina NP, Hall EA, et al. The relative effectiveness of women-only and mixed-gender treatment for substance-abusing women. J Subst Abuse Treat 2011;40(4):336–48.

73. Covington SS. Women and addiction: a trauma-informed approach. J Psychoactive Drugs 2008;40:377–85.

74. Markoff LS, Fallot RD, Reed BG, et al. Implementing trauma-informed alcohol and other drug and mental health services for women: Lessons learned in a multisite demonstration project. Am J Orthopsychiatry 2005;75(4):525–39.

75. Fadus MC, Squeglia LM, Valadez EA, et al. Adolescent substance use disorder treatment: an update on evidence-based strategies. Curr Psychiatry Rep 2019; 21(10):96.

76. Tolou-Shams M, Dauria EF, Folk J, et al. VOICES: an efficacious trauma-informed, gender-responsive cannabis use intervention for justice and school-referred girls with lifetime substance use history. Drug Alcohol Depend 2021;228:108934.

Focusing on Racial, Historical and Intergenerational Trauma, and Resilience

A Paradigm to Better Serving Children and Families

Lisa R. Fortuna, MD, MPH[a],*, Amalia Londoño Tobón, MD[b],
Yohanis Leonor Anglero, MD[c], Alejandra Postlethwaite, MD[d],
Michelle V. Porche, EdD[a], Eugenio M. Rothe, MD[e]

KEYWORDS

- Intergenerational trauma • Racism • Historical trauma • Black • Latinx
- American Indian/Alaska Native (AI/AN) • Children • Resilience

KEY POINTS

- Intergenerational trauma is a term that is used to describe the impact of a traumatic experience or experiences, not only on one generation but also on subsequent generations.
- Racism and structural inequities are drivers of intergenerational trauma that can inflict negative biological, social, and psychological consequences across generations for children and their families, and entire communities.
- Traumatic events that may lead to intergenerational trauma for children include, but are not limited to, direct and indirect exposure to racism and discrimination, parental incarceration, substance use, domestic violence, separations, abuse and neglect, natural disasters, and displacement.
- Along with intergenerational trauma, it is important to consider historical trauma as events which can have a lasting impact on generations.

[a] University of California San Francisco, Zuckerberg San Francisco General Hospital, Department of Psychiatry and Behavioral Sciences, 1001 Potrero Avenue 7M8, San Francisco, CA 94110, USA; [b] National Institutes of Health, National Institute on Minority Health and Health Disparities, 9000 Rockville Pike, Bethesda, MD 20892, USA; [c] Boston Children's Hospital, Children's Hospital, 300 Longwood Avenue, Boston, MA 02115, USA; [d] Neighborhood Healthcare, 13010 Poway Rd. Poway, CA 92064, USA; [e] Herbert Wertheim College of Medicine Florida International University, FIU Health Miami, 11200 Southwest 8th Street, Miami, FL 33199, USA
* Corresponding author.
E-mail address: lisa.fortuna@ucsf.edu
Twitter: @fortuna_lisa (L.R.F.)

Child Adolesc Psychiatric Clin N Am 31 (2022) 237–250
https://doi.org/10.1016/j.chc.2021.11.004
1056-4993/22/© 2021 Elsevier Inc. All rights reserved.

INTRODUCTION

Over the past decade, clinicians and scholars have increasingly studied how psychological trauma is passed down from one generation to the next.[1] Intergenerational trauma is defined as the impact of a traumatic experience(s), not only on one generation but also on subsequent generations[1] (**Box 1** for glossary of important biological, social and psychological terms related to intergenerational trauma). Research across populations demonstrates that intergenerational trauma can have lasting biopsychosocial ramifications. For example, the offspring of trauma survivors are more likely to develop posttraumatic stress disorder (PTSD), mood, and anxiety disorders.[1] This "trauma inheritance" is not only socially transmitted but also biologically embedded.

Intergenerational trauma can be particularly poignant for families that have been traumatized in severe forms (eg, sexual abuse, rape, murder, etc.) and when in the context of historical trauma.[2] Historical trauma refers to multigenerational trauma experienced by a specific cultural, racial or ethnic group that is typically related to major events that oppress and harm a particular group of people.[3] This includes genocides, slavery, colonialism, as well as continued systemic injustices and racism. It is important to note that intergenerational trauma affects groups of individuals in

---

Box 1
Glossary of key clinical terms

- *Intergenerational Trauma:* is the psychological effect that an individual or collective trauma experienced by an individual, group of people, or families has on subsequent generations.

- *Collective Trauma:* traumatic event that is shared by a group of people. It may involve a small group, like a family, or it may involve an entire society. Examples of traumatic events that affect groups may include natural disasters, mass shootings, famine, war, or pandemics.

- *Historical Trauma:* Historical trauma is multigenerational trauma experienced by a specific cultural, racial or ethnic group. It is related to major events that oppressed a particular group of people because of their status as oppressed. Examples of historical trauma include slavery, the Holocaust, forced migrations, and the violent colonization of Native American and Indigenous People?.

- *Epigenetics:* Epigenetics literally means "above" or "on top of" genetics. It refers to external modifications to DNA that turn genes "on" or "off." One example of an epigenetic change is DNA methylation, which alters gene expression, and serves as a biological mechanism for the intergenerational inheritance of the effects of stress.

- *Systemic Racism:* A system (consisting of structures, policies, practices, and norms) that structures opportunity and assigns value based on race and unfairly disadvantages people of color and communities.

- *Racial Trauma:* Racial trauma or race-based traumatic stress is the cumulative effects of racism (often in addition to other adversity) on an individual or group's mental and physical health.

- *Evidence-Based Practice:* Evidence-based practice refers to a clinical decision-making approach for which the practitioner, in consultation with the client "explicitly, conscientiously, and judiciously" selects the evidence-based treatment options best suited to meet the client's needs and obtain optimal outcomes.

- *Dyadic Therapies:* involve treatment delivered to a parent and child simultaneously. Several manualized dyadic approaches have shown evidence of effectiveness in treating social-emotional and behavioral problems and traumatic stress in young children and caregivers, supporting health attachments and development.

different ways, particularly when it is superimposed on historical trauma, current social contexts, and inequities. For example, Black families who have ancestors that were enslaved, emotionally and psychologically experience intergenerational trauma in a different manner than those who are Jewish and have family members affected by the Holocaust, or Native Americans whose great-grandparents were separated from families and forced into cultural assimilation or Latinx and immigrant populations who have experienced displacement from other countries of origin. Therefore, it is crucial to understand the context and particularities of the historical trauma that individuals and families have experienced, and how these intersect with current experiences of adversity and inequity.[3]

The consequences of intergenerational trauma and related social contexts are not usually considered in mental health practice unless a therapist or other mental health professional is oriented to doing so in their assessments and clinical approach. In addition, the existing research on intergenerational trauma has overly focused on individual risk factors and on individual parenting.[1] Although the caregiver–child relationship is important, a focus in this area should not be at the expense of understanding social, structural, and historical context. For example, Black youth are less likely to receive trauma treatment[4] and more like to terminate services early[5] compared with their peers. In contrast, interventions that integrate the social and culturally salient factors related to intergenerational trauma and discrimination have shown better engagement of Black youth and families and also to be clinically effective.[6,7]

In this article, we consider intergenerational and historical trauma, how it affects individuals across generations, and we discuss the implications for child and adolescent development, mental health services, and child-serving systems of care. Although intergenerational and historical trauma have negatively affected many populations globally, in this article, we primarily focus on Black, Latinx/Hispanic, and AI/AN communities in the United States and North America. Specifically, we explore intergenerational trauma from a biopsychosocial perspective, consider the interrelationship of intergenerational trauma with structural inequities, racism, historical trauma and oppression, and identify clinical and systems of care approaches for addressing intergenerational trauma in working with children, adolescents, and families and supporting posttraumatic growth.

THE "Biological EMBEDDING" OF INTERGENERATIONAL TRAUMA

Besides affecting the psychosocial wellbeing of the child, intergenerational and historical trauma can affect physical health through human biology; it is cumulative and reverberates across generations.[8] A large body of research supports the theory of "biological embedding," which refers to biological mechanisms by which adverse or potentially traumatic experiences get "under the skin" of individuals.[9] One of the main biological mechanisms that has been studied is epigenetics. Epigenetics refers to modifications of DNA and histones via biochemical alterations, such as methylation and demethylation that alter gene expression in response to the environment.[10] Findings from epigenetic studies suggest that biological inheritable factors impact the development of offspring independent of and in interaction with perinatal and early childhood direct exposures to stress.[11] Severe stress can induce maternal and offspring disrupted HPA axis regulation, stress regulation,[12] and have also been associated with disruptions in brain structure and activity, autonomic functioning, immune function and inflammation, metabolism, and microbiome functioning.[11] This includes stress stemming from socioeconomic disadvantage, adversity, and racism.[12]

Neurobiological effects such as DNA methylation can exert an effect on brain function over a long-term period and manifest as somatic effects of childhood trauma including disturbances of the stress axis and immune-inflammatory mechanisms, metabolic dysregulation, and risk for mood disorders, anxiety, and PTSD.[13]

These biological mechanisms are at least in part involved in how historically traumatic events such as the Holocaust, affect the offspring of survivors. That is, child descendants of Holocaust survivors not only display trauma symptoms similar to those of their caregivers who experienced the direct traumatic event[14,15] but also have epigenetic modification[16]—including 42 differentially expressed genes (DEGs), most of which are related to immune and endocrine gene network alterations.[17] Similarly, research on Rwandan genocide survivors found epigenetic modifications of the glucocorticoid receptor in women exposed to genocide during pregnancy and their children who were exposed in utero.[18] Studies are also underway to understand the "biological embedding" of stress and trauma in other populations including the Environmental Influences on Children's Health Outcomes (ECHO) Boricua Study of Puerto Rican families, part of a larger National Institutes of Health initiative.

Although research suggests a biological mechanism for intergenerational and historical traumas, much remains to be studied in this area. Specifically, there is a need for understanding if and how interventions can prevent the "biological transmission" of trauma. Additionally, much of the literature has focused on biological mechanisms of intergenerational adversity transmission, yet limited research has focused on intergenerational resilience transmission. Future research will be helpful in conceptualizations of intergenerational and historical trauma to inform clinical work, public health, and prevention.

INTERRELATIONSHIP OF RACIAL, INTERGENERATIONAL, AND HISTORICAL TRAUMA

Intergenerational trauma is related to racial trauma. Both have been documented to have a negative effect on the health and well-being of communities of color, although it is important to have an ecological and biological model for understanding the context for coping with racial stress and trauma.[19] Racial trauma or race-based traumatic stress is the cumulative effect of racism on an individual or group's mental and physical health.[20] As alluded to earlier, intergenerational trauma affects groups of individuals differently. If the impact of systemic oppression and discrimination, both historical and present day, are not addressed in the context of intergenerational trauma, the negative effects of such may continue to disrupt healthy family development. For example, in the context of the United States, many Black families have experienced the trauma of slavery passed down through generations. Forced migration of millions of people from the continent of Africa over the course of 4 centuries was a consequence of the institution of slavery in the Americas, which has been followed by a long legacy of dehumanization, lynching, economic oppression, and other violence.[21] In the context of that legacy of slavery and anti-Black racism, Black parents in the United States (US) continue to face the necessity of having "the talk" to teach their children how to behave when confronted by the police to avoid being killed. Relatedly, witnessing police violence against Black people and other race-related traumatic events on social media has been found to be positively associated with PTSD and depression among Black and Latinx children.[22] Asian American visibility has been obscured by model minority stereotypes, despite a long history of racism, including worker exploitation in building railroads, being sent to internment camps during World War II, and more recent escalation of anti-Asian hate crimes.[23]

Black Americans in the US have endured economic oppression across generations including redlining (discriminatory practice of denying services, typically financial in nature such as mortgages, to residents of certain areas based on skin color) and persistent inequality in access to wealth. Historical redlining, including the U.S. government's 1930s racially discriminatory grading of neighborhoods' mortgage creditworthiness, has been identified as a structural determinant of present-day risk of preterm birth within what continue to be racially segregated neighborhoods.[24] Building on long-standing evidence of greater rates of intergenerational downward mobility for Blacks, Chetty and colleagues[25] used full population tax and Census data to confirm that Black children are more likely than White children to fall below their parents' relative income position. Therefore, the legacy of anti-Black racism perpetuates social and structural inequities, which in turn can contribute to the risk for PTSD, the direct and indirect passing down of physiologic stress across generations.[24,26] Current trauma research is limited by a scarcity of measures that capture the stress associated specifically with race-related events. However, racial discrimination persists as an important driver of intergenerationally transmitted trauma and stress.[20]

Over multiple generations, American Indian Alaskan Native (AI/AN) peoples have endured traumatic events that have had long-lasting consequences for community members. Previous scholarship has identified a broad array of historical events that might contribute to historical trauma in AI/AN communities including forceful eviction, loss of land, and relocation such as the Trail of Tears which involved the resettling of thousands of Native Americans to Oklahoma in 1838.[27] Other traumatic events have targeted communities indirectly through contamination of the physical environment by radioactive dumping and flooding of homelands.[20] Another type of racial trauma that this community was subjected to was the separation of children from families and forceful boarding school attendance due to government-led efforts of cultural assimilation between 1880 and 1930.[29] These schools were designed to enforce forceful cultural assimilation to the American mainstream and the elimination of Native American language and customs. A study conducted by Evans-Campbell et al.[30] found that former boarding school attendees reported higher rates of current illicit drug use and alcohol use disorder and were significantly more likely to have attempted suicide and experienced suicidal thoughts in their lifetime compared with nonattendees. Individuals raised by boarding school attendees were significantly more likely to have a general anxiety disorder, PTSD symptoms, and have suicidal thoughts.

Child and family-serving systems of care continue to evidence disparities in the AI/AN population of the US. In 2019, an estimated 5596 (2%) children entering the foster care system were identified as American Indian or Alaska Native[31] which is an overrepresentation of nearly double that of the general AI/AN child population.[32] In addition, AI/AN children have been found to be the group with the highest rate of entries to the foster care system due to parental substance use.[33]

All these markers serve to highlight the effects of intergenerational trauma combined with present-day disparities. Consequences to these events at the community level have included the breakdown of traditional culture and values and the loss of traditional rites of passage, which contribute to negative health outcomes such as high rates of substance use, high rates of physical illness including obesity, and internalized racism.[28] In a study conducted with elders from 2 large reservation communities, Whitbeck and colleagues[34] explored responses to a variety of historical and contemporary events negatively affecting indigenous people and developed a research scale to measure historical trauma. They found that although respondents were generations removed from these historically traumatic events, the trauma associated with events and the resulting loss of indigenous language in their community, loss of culture, and loss of land was clearly still part of their emotional life; as much as a third of the participants identifying thinking about these topics daily and experiencing associated feelings of anger/avoidance and anxiety and depression.[34] Understanding the effects of historical trauma have led to treatment interventions such as tribal members walking the Trail of Tears to engage experientially with the sense of the place, facilitating healing and changes in health beliefs, attitudes, and behaviors.[27] Studies of university-tribal collaborations have emphasized connections to the land as an important cultural strength on which to build efforts to promote mental health for AI/AN children.[35]

Immigrant families and communities in the United States have faced collective trauma, which is often hidden in the stories of individuals and families who have been displaced.[36] Individuals who migrate from Latin America to the United States and their descendants-are particularly affected by collective and intergenerational trauma due to legacies of colonialism, political violence, and migration-related stressors.[37] There is growing evidence that migration, postmigratory factors, displacement and family separation all can have a negative impact on the mental health of immigrants, refugee, and asylum-seeking individuals, families, and communities.[38] The recent increase in forcible displacement internationally, due to disasters, violence, and political conflicts necessitates understanding the factors associated with immigrant and refugee child mental health.[39] At the writing of this article, Haiti has experienced a recent earthquake, followed by a hurricane, all on the heels of the assassination of the Haitian president and political upheaval. This is in the context of a previous devastating earthquake disaster in 2010, preexisting poverty, a legacy of slavery, anti-Black racism experienced by the diaspora, centuries of colonialism, and environmental injustice. Immigrant populations from other countries, including Latin America, have histories of experiencing their own historical and multigenerational trauma based on political violence, disasters, and other national collective trauma, which contributes to forced migration.[40]

Premigration trauma is recognized as a key predictor of mental health outcomes in immigrants, refugees, and asylum seekers. Many recent immigration policies aim to deter migration at the Mexican border or to increase deportations from the US. These have resulted in a growing number of family separations and unaccompanied minors on the U.S. southern border. The multigenerational effects of these laws that target immigrants are illustrated in Vignette 1.

Research has also increasingly focused on the psychological effects of postmigration stressors in the host country including poverty and discrimination.[41] In the US, children of immigrant families are embedded in interdependent intergenerational relationships, which affect their mental health outcomes.[42] Gulbas and colleagues[43] found that the U.S. born immigrant children of undocumented parents have elevated risk for developing depression, anxiety, and learning difficulties, triggered by the deportation of a parent, or the threat of parental deportation. In addition, youth who were brought to the US as minors by their migrant families face their own risk of deportation. The Deferred Action for Childhood Arrivals (DACA) is a U.S. immigration policy, which could allow some individuals who arrived in the US as children to receive a renewable 2-year period of deferred action from deportation and become eligible for a work permit, and to access higher education.[44] The young people to whom this applies, called Dreamers, have emerged as important voices as activists working not only for the benefit of their own plight but also that of their parents and undocumented communities, and exemplify a potential source of resistance in the face of uncertainty following threats to DACA policies.[44] Dreamer college students experience greater stress overload, more mental health symptoms, and worse grades than their documented peers.[44]

An appreciation of intergenerational trauma as experienced in diverse populations is important not only for understanding vulnerabilities and risk but also for resilience. Cultivating opportunities for communities to respond and heal from past and current experiences are important for addressing intergenerational trauma sequelae.[45] Posttraumatic growth is defined by improvements in traumatic stress in the areas of self-perception, relationships, and outlook on life after traumatic experiences.[46] Over the past 3 decades, investigations have reported posttraumatic growth after various categories of accidental traumas including natural disasters, chronic and acute health problems, transportation accidents, interpersonal and intergenerational traumatic experiences.[47] Many of the interventions which may be helpful in supporting posttraumatic growth in children support them in relationships, include culture and spirituality and include constructing a comprehensive self-narrative that identifies their personal strengths and growth experiences—but much more research is needed.[46]

PREVENTION INTERVENTIONS

Prevention is the most effective intervention approach for the intergenerational transmission of trauma. Prevention requires trauma-specific Interventions with adults and attachment-focused interventions within families. These strategies need to target individual, relationship, familial, community, and societal levels and require a multi-pronged and multisystemic approach. A prime time for prevention is during pregnancy and early childhood. These developmental periods have been shown to be particularly sensitive to environmental adverse and positive experiences.[10] A range of critical developmental processes between parents and children take place during this time. Several studies have demonstrated that both prevention and treatment interventions that take a dyadic approach have lasting outcomes for offspring and caregivers[48] and may lead to economic benefits.[49,50]

One of the prevention interventions that has been shown to be effective is comprehensive early home visiting, a multigenerational, multi-pronged approach that has been described by the Centers for Disease Control and Prevention as one of the most effective ways to ameliorate intergenerational adversity.[51] Variations of comprehensive early home visiting exist but they typically focus on improving the caregiver-child relationship by focusing on the physical and emotional wellbeing of families and access to the necessary resources that they may need. Many of these prevention programs have been tested with populations that have limited access to care, are low-income, and/or are marginalized in other ways. Comprehensive home-visiting interventions improve outcomes in several areas including child health, development, maternal-health, positive parenting practices, family economic self-sufficiency, successful linkages, and referrals, and decreases in child maltreatment, delinquency, family violence, and crime.[52,53]

An example of a comprehensive early home-visiting intervention developed using community participatory strategies with low-income Latinx and Black families, is the *Minding the Baby* (MTB). MTB uses a relational-based approach to meet the specific needs of families. To date, studies with this method show positive intervention effects on child attachment, child health, and parenting.[54,55] Additionally, many years after the intervention, children in the MTB had lower problematic behaviors, lower inflammatory biomarker profiles, and the intervention moderated the relationship between maternal experiences of discrimination and child inflammatory marker levels.[56–58]

The perinatal and early childhood period offers a unique life-course opportunity not only for parental and child prevention of child traumatic stress but also for treatment. Interventions such as Child-Parent Psychotherapy (CPP)[59] and Pregnancy-Child-Parent Psychotherapy[60] have demonstrated the efficacy and effectiveness of taking a dyadic, relational focused, trauma, and culturally informed approach to treating families who have been exposed to trauma. Additionally, these interventions encourage clinicians to not only understand the current traumatic experience but also the multi-generational and historical trauma that families may have endured, past supports, coping and strengths, and how these all may relate to both current trauma and opportunity for healing. The focus on the relationship as a vehicle for healing is at the core of CPP and similar interventions.

EVIDENCE-BASED APPROACHES

Most trauma therapy interventions target individual-level factors (eg, coping skills), rather than systemic factors (eg, stressors in the social environment). Therapies that focus on general coping strategies for healing from interpersonal trauma (eg, diaphragmatic breathing) may also ignore culturally specific strategies essential to addressing trauma for African American and other youth of color.[6] Metzger and colleagues[7] integrated racial socialization—a culturally relevant and commonly practiced familial coping strategy—into trauma-focused cognitive behavioral therapy (TF-CBT) to improve trauma-related outcomes among African American youth. The racial socialization messages are integrated into the CBT, including racial pride messages about African American culture and heritage, navigating barriers based on discrimination and racism including managing social interactions between African Americans and majority populations on individual, cultural, and institutional levels, equality, and achievement.[61] The intervention includes caregivers exploring these themes with their child, along with cognitive therapy and emotional regulation skills, which support both the child and family system.[62] Interventions which consider faith and spirituality as key sources of resilience can be helpful for many Black, Latinx and immigrant families.[63] The importance of cultural practices, spirituality, and group identity are shared elements in an intervention aimed at helping youth to heal from intergenerational, historical, and racial trauma.[64,65]

Trauma-informed approaches that are responsive to structural and social inequities are also important for healing. Through their interactions with medical systems, families may experience triggers that are retraumatizing. A recent review by Alvarez[66] found that experiences of implicit and explicit discrimination in schools and inequities in the quality of education can shape students' experiences with traumatic stress. Systems and schools can shift that discourse by building anti-racist consciousness, supporting trauma-exposed youth and families, and curtailing institutionally induced trauma and experiences of implicit and explicit trauma across generations.

SUMMARY

Clinical systems which focus on treating solely presenting symptoms such as anxiety and depression without consideration to social and generational contexts have less chance of success, especially among marginalized communities. Integrating and prioritizing the values and practices of communities is a key factor and effective interventions are child and family-centered, often dyadic, and always socio-contextually informed. For example, traditional healing methods, commitment to the wellness of tribal communities, spiritual practices and beliefs, relationships with elders and ceremonial practices, have been important for healing in AI/AN peoples.[67] Most medical models for treating traumatic stress reflect limited understandings of the sociopolitical, intergenerational, and historical context of trauma for communities of color. Furthermore, the emphasis of Western mental health services fails to recognize the importance of emic understandings of locally resonant coping strategies for healing. However, effective treatment of children, adolescents, and families includes an in-depth understanding of cultural processes through which healing occurs and is maintained.

CLINICS CARE POINTS

- Overall, the research on evidence-based prevention interventions highlights the following key ingredients for supporting families exposed to adversity and trauma:
  - 1. relational (ie, focus on the caregiver-child relationship)
  - 2. tailored to the specific needs of families including cultural responsiveness
  - 3. use a dyadic and multigenerational approach
  - 4. focus on emotional and physical health
  - 5. are trauma informed.

- Providers should recognize that cultural, racial, and ethnic groups are heterogeneous, and not every member of a group has the same response to a current or past traumatic event. Taking time to ask about family history and experiences is an important part of assessment.

- Child and family-serving systems of care working with members of underserved cultural groups can help by gaining a fuller understanding of the clients' historical and community's context of both trauma and healing practices.

- Providers can seek and build alliances with local, respected individuals such as pastors and community leaders, tribal leaders in AI/AN populations as part of treatment, and for understanding the contextual factors that impact intergenerational trauma.

- The use of clinically proven evidence-based treatments such as Child and Parent Psychotherapy (Dyadic models in early childhood) and Trauma-Focused CBT that also integrates culturally salient coping practices and beliefs can better engage families and result in good outcomes.

VIGNETTE 1: MARIA'S STORY

Maria is a 16-year-old girl from Michoacán, Mexico who has been living in a shelter in Tijuana for the last 2 months. She left Michoacán with her mother and siblings fleeing the violence of the drug cartels. The family is hoping to be granted asylum in the US. Maria's family has experienced generations of labor exploitation as people who live in poverty. Maria was seen at a volunteer behavioral support service at an immigration shelter. She was experiencing PTSD-related symptoms which included flashbacks, nightmares, difficulties consolidating sleep, avoidance, extreme dysphoria, crying spells, and intermittent suicidal ideation. These are partly related to a history of sexual and physical abuse at the hands of her biological father. She recently disclosed this to her mother. Maria believes that her mother may be minimizing her abuse because several women in her family, including her mother, have also suffered from sexual or physical abuse by other family members. These have all been unspoken topics in the family. Maria has been pinching herself with the hopes that physical pain will dull her emotional pain. A bilingual, bicultural volunteer provided her with relaxation techniques and referred her to psychotherapy to be provided by mental health volunteers of a humanitarian organization. They agreed that engaging her mother as part of treatment, once Maria feels ready, would be important. Once Maria and her mother were safely resettled in the US, they were connected to an immigrant serving and led agency that offered social support, access to legal resources and provided vocational and economic opportunities for Maria's mother. Attending to these needs provided further opportunities for healing. Ongoing therapy, for both Maria and her mother further deepened the exploration of their family's intergenerational trauma and pain. The dyadic family-focused care integrated cultural traditions and other sources of strength that Maria and her mother could share together. This contributed significantly to improving their relationship, coping, and healing.

VIGNETTE 2: ESTHER

Esther is a 16-year-old girl from Haiti who presented for an inpatient psychiatric admission for the second time in the past year due to suicidal ideation. She had an extensive trauma history in her early childhood including neglect and failure to properly provide medical care for her Sickle Cell Disease. Her mother, who was also medically ill, died from the same condition. Esther was 5 years old during a massive earthquake in Haiti that displaced her family. She lives with an aunt and has expressed difficulties adapting to being a Black person in a predominantly white community and school where she now resides. She explains that it is difficult to make friends, that she does not like her body, and that she is constantly comparing her physical appearance to the other girls in her school. Esther reports ongoing flashbacks and nightmares and wishes she were dead like others in her family, stating she feels guilty that she was the one who survived instead of them. She also began to have somatic symptoms in the form of nonepileptic seizures. In therapy, she began to work on a trauma narrative, which explored her past experiences, and was offered techniques on how to help cope with distress. She and her aunt were referred for family-based psychotherapy helping them understand not only her individual trauma but also an opportunity to consider collective and racial trauma as an immigrant to the US. The providers were also able to connect Esther to a community-based organization, started during the Haitian HIV crisis some decades ago, which supports Haitian youth who have experienced trauma and loss. The organization uses instruction in traditional Haitian music and arts and classical music as expressive therapy and a means to offer connection with other youth and supportive adults, promoting healthy youth development, including healthy racial identity.

VIGNETTE 3: MARS

Mars is a 14-year-old Black youth who goes by they/them pronouns who was admitted to the hospital due to aggression in the home toward their brother and grandmother. Mars started having increased irritability and aggressive outbursts after their father was incarcerated 2 years ago due to charges of domestic violence and sexual assault toward Mars' sister. Mars refused to talk about their father with the treatment team. Mars engaged in some processing of their aggression and their trauma and started showing symptoms of major depressive disorder when they learned that they may be removed from their mother's custody because of the aggression they had engaged in against siblings at home. Eventually, Mars was referred to a program for children with history of trauma where they could continue to process the trauma they witnessed as a young child, the loss of their father, and also practice skills for regulating their emotions. Mars' mother, siblings, and grandmother were part of the therapy. The therapist was skillful in exploring the family's trauma narrative including the racial inequities and cumulative losses they had all experienced, and helped the family consider their strengths, which could be brought forward to assist Mars. Mars and their family continued work with a community agency that offered a family partner, an African American woman with lived experience who helped the family navigate services and connect to supports.

DISCLOSURE

Dr. Londoño Tobón performed this work while completing a post-doctoral fellowship at Lifespan/Brown University (T32 MH019927). She is now supported by the Division of Intramural Research, National Institute of Minority Health and Health Disparities, National Institutes of Health. The contents and views in this manuscript are those of the authors and should not be construed to represent the views of the National Institutes of Health. Dr. Fortuna, Dr. Anglero, Dr. Postlethwaite. Dr. Porche and Dr. Roth have nothing to disclose.

REFERENCES

1. Cerdeña JP, Rivera LM, Spak JM. Intergenerational trauma in Latinxs: a scoping review. Soc Sci Med 2021;270:113662.
2. O'Neill L, Fraser T, Kitchenham A, et al. Hidden burdens: a review of intergenerational, historical and complex trauma, implications for indigenous families. J Child Adolesc Trauma 2018;11(2):173–86.
3. Kirmayer LJ, Gone JP, Moses J. Rethinking historical trauma. Transcult Psychiatry 2014;51(3):299–319.
4. Merikangas KR, He JP, Burstein M, et al. Service utilization for lifetime mental disorders in U.S. adolescents: results of tho National Comorbidity Survey-Adolescent Supplement (NCS-A). J Am Acad Child Adolesc Psychiatry 2011; 50(1):32–45.
5. Lester K, Resick PA, Young-Xu Y, et al. Impact of race on early treatment termination and outcomes in posttraumatic stress disorder treatment. J Consult Clin Psychol 2010;78(4):480–9.
6. Anderson RE, Jones S, Anyiwo N, et al. What's race got to do with it? racial socialization's contribution to Black adolescent coping. J Res Adolesc 2019; 29(4):822–31.
7. Metzger IW, Anderson RE, Are F, et al. Healing interpersonal and racial trauma: integrating racial socialization into trauma-focused cognitive behavioral therapy for African American youth. Child Maltreat 2021;26(1):17–27.
8. Evans TA, Erwin JA. Retroelement-derived RNA and its role in the brain. Semin Cell Dev Biol 2021;114:68–80.
9. McEwen BS. Brain on stress: how the social environment gets under the skin. Proc Natl Acad Sci U S A 2012;109(Suppl 2):17180–5.
10. Londono Tobon A, Diaz Stransky A, Ross DA, et al. Effects of maternal prenatal stress: mechanisms, implications, and novel Therapeutic interventions. Biol Psychiatry 2016;80(11):e85–7.
11. Berens AE, Jensen SKG, Nelson CA. Biological embedding of childhood adversity: from physiological mechanisms to clinical implications. BMC Med 2017; 15(1):135.
12. Scorza P, Duarte CS, Hipwell AE, et al. Research Review: intergenerational transmission of disadvantage: epigenetics and parents' childhoods as the first exposure. J Child Psychol Psychiatry 2019;60(2):119–32.
13. Jaworska-Andryszewska P, Rybakowski JK. Childhood trauma in mood disorders: Neurobiological mechanisms and implications for treatment. Pharmacol Rep 2019;71(1):112–20.

14. Rakoff V, Sigal JJ, Epstein NB. Children and families of concentration camp survivors. Canada's Ment Health 1966;14(4):24–6.

15. Sigal JJ, Weinfeld M. Trauma and rebirth: intergenerational effects of the Holocaust. New York, NY, England: Praeger Publishers; 1989.

16. Yehuda R, Daskalakis NP, Bierer LM, et al. Holocaust exposure induced intergenerational effects on FKBP5 methylation. Biol Psychiatry 2016;80(5):372–80.

17. Daskalakis NP, Xu C, Bader HN, et al. Intergenerational trauma is associated with expression alterations in glucocorticoid- and immune-related genes. Neuropsychopharmacology 2021;46(4):763–73.

18. Perroud N, Rutembesa E, Paoloni-Giacobino A, et al. The Tutsi genocide and transgenerational transmission of maternal stress: epigenetics and biology of the HPA axis. World J Biol Psychiatry 2014;15(4):334–45.

19. Saleem FT, Anderson RE, Williams M. Addressing the "Myth" of racial trauma: developmental and ecological considerations for youth of color. Clin Child Fam Psychol Rev 2020;23(1):1–14.

20. Kirkinis K, Pieterse AL, Martin C, et al. Racism, racial discrimination, and trauma: a systematic review of the social science literature. Ethn Health 2021;26(3): 392–412.

21. Gomez MA. African identity and slavery in the Americas. Radic Hist Rev 1999;(75):111–20.

22. Tynes BM, Willis HA, Stewart AM, et al. Race-related traumatic events online and mental health among adolescents of color. J Adolesc Health 2019;65(3):371–7.

23. Yip T, Cheah CSL, Kiang L, et al. Rendered invisible: are Asian Americans a model or a marginalized minority? Am Psychol 2021;76(4):575–81.

24. Krieger N, Van Wye G, Huynh M, et al. Structural racism, historical redlining, and risk of preterm birth in New York City, 2013-2017. Am J Public Health 2020;110(7): 1046–53.

25. Chetty R, Hendren N, Jones MR, et al. Race and economic opportunity in the United States: an intergenerational perspective. Q J Econ 2019;135(2):711–83.

26. Hampton-Anderson JN, Carter S, Fani N, et al. Adverse childhood experiences in African Americans: framework, practice, and policy. Am Psychol 2021;76(2): 314–25.

27. Schultz K, Walters KL, Beltran R, et al. I'm stronger than I thought": Native women reconnecting to body, health, and place. Health Place 2016;40:21–8.

28. Evans-Campbell T. Historical trauma in American Indian/Native Alaska communities: a multilevel framework for exploring impacts on individuals, families, and communities. J Interpers Violence 2008;23(3):316–38.

29. Enoch MA, Albaugh BJ. Review: genetic and environmental risk factors for alcohol use disorders in American Indians and Alaskan Natives. Am J Addict 2017;26(5):461–8.

30. Evans-Campbell T, Walters KL, Pearson CR, et al. Indian boarding school experience, substance use, and mental health among urban two-spirit American Indian/Alaska natives. Am J Drug Alcohol Abuse 2012;38(5):421–7.

31. U.S. Department of Health and Human Services. The AFCARS report. Washington, DC: Children's Bureau; 2020.

32. Landers AL, Danes SM, Campbell AR, et al. Abuse after abuse: the recurrent maltreatment of American Indian children in foster care and adoption. Child Abuse Negl 2021;111:104805.

33. Meinhofer A, Onuoha E, Angleró-Díaz Y, et al. Parental drug use and racial and ethnic disproportionality in the U.S. foster care system. Child Youth Serv Rev 2020;118.

34. Whitbeck LB, Adams GW, Hoyt DR, et al. Conceptualizing and measuring historical trauma among American Indian people. Am J Community Psychol 2004; 33(3–4):119–30.
35. Goodkind JR, Gorman B, Hess JM, et al. Reconsidering culturally competent approaches to American Indian healing and well-being. Qual Health Res 2015; 25(4):486–99.
36. Thomas SL, Thomas SD. Displacement and health. Br Med Bull 2004;69:115–27.
37. Fortuna LR, Porche MV, Alegria M. Political violence, psychosocial trauma, and the context of mental health services use among immigrant Latinos in the United States. Ethn Health 2008;13(5):435–63.
38. Li SS, Liddell BJ, Nickerson A. The relationship between post-migration stress and psychological disorders in refugees and asylum Seekers. Curr Psychiatry Rep 2016;18(9):82.
39. Kamimura A, Weaver S, Sin K, et al. Immigration stress among refugees resettled in the United States. Int J Soc Psychiatry 2021;67(2):144–9.
40. Cénat JM, McIntee SE, Blais-Rochette C. Symptoms of posttraumatic stress disorder, depression, anxiety and other mental health problems following the 2010 earthquake in Haiti: a systematic review and meta-analysis. J Affect Disord 2020;273:55–85.
41. Rothe EM, Pumariega AJ. Immigration, cultural identity, and mental health: Psycho-social Implications of the reshaping of America. New York, NY, US: Oxford University Press; 2020.
42. Zayas LH, Aguilar-Gaxiola S, Yoon H, et al. The distress of citizen-children with detained and deported parents. J Child Fam Stud 2015;24(11):3213–23.
43. Gulbas LE, Zayas LH, Yoon H, et al. Deportation experiences and depression among U.S. citizen-children with undocumented Mexican parents. Child Care Health Dev 2016;42(2):220–30.
44. Amirkhan JH, Velasco SE. Stress overload and the new nightmare for Dreamers. J Am Coll Health 2021;69(1):67–73.
45. Narayan AJ, Rivera LM, Bernstein RE, et al. Positive childhood experiences predict less psychopathology and stress in pregnant women with childhood adversity: a pilot study of the benevolent childhood experiences (BCEs) scale. Child Abuse Negl 2018;78:19–30.
46. Vloet TD, Vloet A, Bürger A, et al. Post-traumatic growth in children and adolescents. J Trauma Stress Disor Treat 2017;6(4):1–7.
47. Sheridan G, Carr A. Survivors' lived experiences of posttraumatic growth after institutional childhood abuse: an interpretative phenomenological analysis. Child Abuse Negl 2020;103:104430.
48. Karoly LA, Greenwood PW, Sohler Everingham SM, et al. Early childhood interventions: benefits, Costs, and Savings. Santa Monica, CA: RAND Corporation; 1998.
49. Minkovitz CS, Hughart N, Strobino D, et al. A practice-based intervention to enhance quality of care in the first 3 years of life: the Healthy Steps for Young Children Program. Jama 2003;290(23):3081–91.
50. Minkovitz CS, Strobino D, Mistry KB, et al. Healthy Steps for young children: sustained results at 5.5 Years. Pediatrics 2007;120(3):e658.
51. Garner AS. Home visiting and the biology of toxic stress: opportunities to address early childhood adversity. Pediatrics 2013;132(Suppl 2):S65–73.
52. Molloy C, Beatson R, Harrop C, et al. Systematic review: effects of sustained nurse home visiting programs for disadvantaged mothers and children. J Adv Nurs 2021;77(1):147–61.

53. Sama-Miller E, Akers L, Mraz-Esposito A, et al. Home Visiting Evidence of Effectiveness Review: Executive Summary. Office of Planning, Research and Evaluation, Administration for Children and Families, US: Department of Health and Human Services. Washington, DC; 2018.

54. Sadler LS, Slade A, Close N, et al. Minding the Baby: Enhancing reflectiveness to improve early health and relationship outcomes in an interdisciplinary home visiting program. Infant Ment Health J 2013;34(5):391–405.

55. Slade A, Holland ML, Ordway MR, et al. Minding the Baby®: Enhancing parental reflective functioning and infant attachment in an attachment-based, interdisciplinary home visiting program. Dev Psychopathol 2020;32(1):123–37.

56. Condon EM, Londono Tobon A, Jackson B, et al. Maternal experiences of racial discrimination, child Indicators of toxic stress, and the Minding the Baby early home visiting intervention. Nurse Res 2021;70(5S Suppl 1):S43–52.

57. Londono Tobon A, Condon E, Slade, A., Holland M, Mayes L, Sadler L. Effects of an Attachment-Based Home Visiting Intervention on Inflammatory Biomarkers among Multiethnic Children living in Underserved Communities. in preparation.

58. Londono Tobon A, Condon E, Sadler LS, et al. School age effects of Minding the Baby—an attachment-based home-visiting intervention—on parenting and child behaviors. Dev Psychopathology 2020;1–13.

59. Lieberman AF, Ghosh Ippen C, VANH P. Child-parent psychotherapy: 6-month follow-up of a randomized controlled trial. J Am Acad Child Adolesc Psychiatry 2006;45(8):913–8.

60. Lieberman AF, Diaz MA, Castro G, et al. Make room for baby: perinatal child-parent psychotherapy to repair trauma and promote attachment. Guilford Publications; 2020.

61. Hughes D, Rodriguez J, Smith EP, et al. Parents' ethnic-racial socialization practices: a review of research and directions for future study. Dev Psychol 2006; 42(5):747–70.

62. Duarté-Vélez Y, Gomez J, Jiménez Colón G, et al. Socio-cognitive behavioral therapy for suicidal behavior with a Puerto Rican Male adolescent. Evidence-based Pract Child Adolesc Ment Health 2018;3(2):81–97.

63. Stevenson HC Jr, Cameron R, Herrero-Taylor T, et al. Development of the Teenager experience of racial socialization scale: Correlates of race-related socialization frequency from the perspective of Black youth. J Black Psychol 2002; 28(2):84–106.

64. Hernandez JA. Family-centered culture care: Touched by an Angel. J Clin Ethics 2019;30(4):376–83.

65. Allen J, Wexler L, Rasmus S. Protective Factors as a Unifying Framework for Strength-Based Intervention and Culturally Responsive American Indian and Alaska Native Suicide Prevention. Prevention Science: the Official Journal of the Society for Prevention Research. 2021 Jun. DOI: 10.1007/s11121-021-01265-0. PMID: 34169406.

66. Alvarez A. Seeing race in the research on youth trauma and education: a critical review. Rev Educ Res 2020;90(5):583–626.

67. Ramirez LC, Hammack PL. Surviving colonization and the quest for healing: narrative and resilience among California Indian tribal leaders. Transcultural Psychiatry 2014;51(1):112–33.

Cultural and Structural Humility and Addressing Systems of Care Disparities in Mental Health Services for Black, Indigenous, and People of Color Youth

Annie Sze Yan Li, MD[a],*, Qortni Lang, MD[a], Jang Cho, MD[b],
Vinh-Son Nguyen, MD[c], Shankar Nandakumar, MD[c]

KEYWORDS

- Cultural humility • Racism • Mental health • Disparities

KEY POINTS

- Cultural humility is an active, dynamic approach for health care professionals to cultivate awareness, knowledge, and understanding of their patients from diverse cultural and ethnic backgrounds.
- Reducing mental health care disparities requires the recognition of how racism and discrimination impact the mental health well-being of Black, Indigenous, and People of Color (BIPOC) youths.
- The incorporation of culture and structural humility in clinical care, medical training, and professional development programs can lead to increased engagement, mutual respect, and understanding and help to bridge gaps, reduce disparities, and promote healing.

INTRODUCTION

In 2003, the Institute of Medicine (IOM) published findings and evidence showing the existence of differences in how people of color receive health care in the United States. The volume. titled *Unequal Treatment*, examines the myriad of ways in which

[a] NYU Grossman School of Medicine, NYU Langone Health, NYC Health + Hospital - Bellevue Medical Center, NYU Child Study Center, One Park Avenue, 7th Floor, New York, NY 10016, USA; [b] Cultivate Psychiatry 420 S 72nd Avenue, #180-346 Yakima, WA 98908, USA; [c] Menninger Department of Psychiatry and Behavioral Sciences, Lee and Joe Jamail Specialty Care Center, 1977 Butler Boulevard, Houston, TX 77030, USA
* Corresponding author.
E-mail address: Annie.Li@nyulangone.org

Child Adolesc Psychiatric Clin N Am 31 (2022) 251–259
https://doi.org/10.1016/j.chc.2021.11.003
1056-4993/22/© 2021 Elsevier Inc. All rights reserved.

race and ethnicity impacts care access, care delivery, and the quality of care.[1] Such differences are recognized as disparities and are rooted in racial and ethnic inequality.

In recent years, there is growing data to identify such disparities in mental health services in Black, Indigenous, and People of Color (BIPOC). When comparing racial and ethnic minorities to the white population, those who belong to minoritized groups have less access to mental health services, are not likely to get needed care, and receive lower quality of care.[2] Between 2015 and 2019, it is estimated that on average, White adolescents ages 12 to 17 were more likely to receive mental health services in a specialty setting (17.2%) than for Hispanic (13.2%), Black (11.8%), and Asian (9.5%) adolescents.[3] Looking at treatment of major depressive disorders alone in the adolescent population, the SAMHSA Center for Behavioral Health Statistics and Quality found that estimates of adolescents who received treatment were higher among White adolescents (46.0%) than among their Black, Hispanic, and Asian counterparts (36.3, 35.6, and 26.2%, respectively).[3]

There are many aspects of the health care environment that influence how historically marginalized groups receive mental health care in the United States. These include, and are not limited to, the historical evolution of health care for BIPOC, systemic discriminatory practices, the current landscape of financial payers and care reimbursement (private v private insurances), health care organizational infrastructure (for-profit vs public/municipal facilities, etc.), the settings in which care is delivered (medical facilities, schools, correctional facilities, home based), and the demographics of the workforce providing care.[1] These factors may, both independently and collectively, influence the quality and level of care that minoritized individuals receive.

It is more openly recognized now that there are inherent aspects of the clinical encounter contributing to health care disparities. How a clinician's attitude, expectations, and behavior in relation to a patient's racial and ethnic origin, along with a patient's own perceptions of a clinician of a particular cultural background, can affect and compromise the care delivering and care receiving process.[1] Both implicit and explicit biases, along with stereotypes, may amplify and perpetuate discriminatory attitudes between the clinician and the patient that contribute to health disparities. Over the years, the emphasis on developing an awareness of biases in the professional setting has been lauded as necessary interventions to address disparities and promote mental health equity.

In this paper, the authors aim to review the concepts of cultural competence and cultural and structural humility, highlight how building racial, ethnic, and cultural awareness in the health care setting can bridge gaps, and present two models currently in existence for which cultural and structural humility are promoted as measures to address ongoing mental health disparities for BIPOC youths in child and adolescent psychiatry.

The Shift from Cultural Competence to Cultural Humility

Cultural competency stemmed from the recognition that to serve a growing and diverse patient population in the United States, clinicians need to be equipped with skills and knowledge about cultures that would help with care delivery. It has been the standard framework for which medical training and curricula building in multiculturalism were based on. Its intentions were to empower both health care systems and professionals to understand the cultures, values, languages, and customs of their patients. Through acquiring such knowledge, attitudes/beliefs, and skills about various cultures, health care professionals and institutions would be better informed to provide care and take part in a respectful patient–clinician relationship.[4]

Over the years, there has been a shift to a different paradigm, one which Trevalon and Murray Garcia proposed as more optimal than cultural competence. The new paradigm promotes a commitment and a lifelong pursuit of engagement, exploration, self-reflection, and self-critique of awareness to and understanding of a patient's cultural background. Termed as cultural humility, it is an experiential process that builds toward mutually respectful and dynamic relationships with patients, communities, colleagues, and themselves.[5]

Trevalon and Murray-Garcia's proposal for cultural humility stems from the recognition that the model of cultural competence has its limitations and pitfalls. First, cultural competence training is highly variable in time and depth, ranging from month-long curricula in medical school and training programs to a yearly video module as part of hospital onboarding. Second, completion of such training may foster a false sense of confidence in clinicians who may equate their own mastery of information about a culture to exert power over the patient, and further stereotype the patient's experience while ignoring potential insight imparted from patients themselves and other parties.[5] Even when integrated into standardized testing, it is not enough to equate memorization of culture-bound syndromes as being culturally competent. Third, an increase in a clinician's attitude, knowledge, and skills of a patient's culture has not consistently demonstrated an improvement in patient satisfaction, health outcome, or reduction in disparities.[6] The expectation for a clinician to be fully versed in the knowledge of all existing cultures is simply unrealistic. Culture is dynamic and ever evolving, and with the growing intersectionality of identities of any one individual, cultural competency limits a comprehensive understanding of the multi-cultural and multi-dimensional nature of the patients we serve. Fluency in a stagnant set of knowledge about a culture may inadvertently box someone into a single group, without taking into consideration the heterogeneity inherent with intersectionality. We can appreciate a better delineation of cultural competence and cultural humility in **Fig. 1**.

Cultural humility facilitates respect and appreciation for diversity that is active, multifaceted, and enriching. Embracing this approach on a structural level is equally critical In evaluating and resolving systemic practices that may contribute to mental health disparities at large. Without an active process of inquiry, it is easy to default to the

Cultural Competence	Cultural Humility
• Finite, has an endpoint. • Fixed, static, unchanging body of knowledge shared by all members of an identified group • "Mastery" conveys Paternalism • Pitfall: "Self proclaimed cultural expert"[4] → perpetuates stereotypes • Does not take into account of intersectionality - (i.e. Chinese-American immigrant, queer woman)	• Dynamic, Lifelong Process • Commitment • Active learning and ongoing engagement through interactions with patients, communities, with themselves • Balanced dynamic between clinician and patient • Reflective practitioner - self appraisal, self critique • Respectful, non paternalistic

Fig. 1. Cultural competence versus cultural humility. (*Data from* Tervalon M, Murray-García J. Cultural humility versus cultural competence: a critical distinction in defining physician training outcomes in multicultural education. J Health Care Poor Underserved. 1998 May;9(2):117-25.)

status quo, which would be a system originally designed from the unilateral perspective of the dominant race and culture. As Metzl and Hansen suggest, clinicians not only require skills that will help them treat patients, they also need to recognize how social and economic determinants, biases, inequities, and blind spots shape health and illness long before the clinician or patients enter the room.[7] The concept of structural humility calls for health professionals to not be complicit in the system in which they train and work. It challenges one to call into question aspects of the infrastructure that perpetuates disparities and moves the dial to affect change toward inclusivity and equity.

CONSIDERATIONS
Cultural Humility in Reducing Care Disparities

How can cultural humility facilitate therapeutic relationship building that potentially results in higher patient satisfaction and engagement in the mental health field? There has been growing evidence to support improvement in the therapeutic alliance when clinicians adopt an element of humility to understand their patients. A 4-tiered study conducted by Hook and colleagues on a therapist's multicultural orientation and cultural humility found that a patient's perception of their therapist as having high cultural humility was associated with two outcomes: high therapeutic working alliance and patients' self-reporting of improvement in therapy.[4] In a subsequent study, Hook and his team looked at cultural humility and incidence of racial microaggressions perpetrated by clinicians. Patients who perceived their therapists as cultivating high cultural humility found these therapists less likely to commit racial microaggressions.[8] When clinicians did commit acts of racial microaggressions, those transgressions were better tolerated when patients perceived their therapists as having high cultural humility. The presumption is that therapists with high cultural humility were more likely able to acknowledge their wrongdoing, appraise oneself, recover from the mishap, and repair the trust and alliance in the patient–therapist relationship.[8]

Looking at another setting for youths, one can appreciate the positive impact of cultural humility in the mentoring program called reVision in the Harris County Juvenile Probation Department in Houston, Texas. This qualitative study looking at how cultural humility influenced mentoring outcomes analyzed the relationships of mentors who were predominantly white, middle to upper class, to their mentees who were predominantly men, LAtinX justice involved youths.[9] It looked at mentors' approach to their mentoring relationships and their capacity to bridge the racial gap with their mentees. Successful mentoring relationships were more likely to occur when mentors initiated connections with a nonjudgmental stance, highlighted the similarities and differences between themselves and the mentees, and attempted to explore and learn the lived experiences and traumas of the delinquent youths.[9] Mentors who understood the lives of their mentees appreciated how family and society factors, including racism, discrimination, poverty and social inequality, perpetuated behaviors of delinquency in these youths. Their enhanced awareness and consciousness of systemic barriers that negatively affect the youths in the juvenile justice system promoted greater engagement in social justice causes. Mentors entered the mentoring relationship with a cultivation of cultural humility. The positive outcome included mentors reporting greater satisfaction in the mentoring experience and mentees' capacity to build trust and positive attachments toward self-improvement.[9]

The capacity of a mental health care professional to develop self-consciousness when working with diverse youths and families is vital. Acknowledgment and incorporation of the family into the treatment of any child is a fundamental part of the field, and relatedly the work of developing structural competence involves understanding how a family system intersects with many other larger systems and not in isolation.[7] As the United States continues to reckon with the pervasiveness of racism in our society, which was further highlighted with the COVID pandemic and recurrent incidents of violence toward BIPOC communities, mental health professionals need to be prepared to enter therapeutic relationships with BIPOC youths. Providers need to open themselves to communicating with families to identify and discuss the impact of racism and discrimination on their mental health. These skills need to be introduced early in professional training and ongoing advocacy enacted to promote these initiatives. Despite the recognition that this work is essential, there are existing barriers that impede this pathway including: (1) inadequate organizational support and training, (2) Ongoing reluctance and avoidance of discussions related to race and racism, (3) prioritizing of medical knowledge and clinical skills in the curriculum over professional interpersonal effectiveness, and (4) resistance and defensiveness in individuals to be challenged on their personal biases.[10]

Health care institutions' commitment to diversity, inclusion, and equity need to include prioritizing professional development of cultural awareness, challenging clinicians to realize their own personal biases, and creating an environment that is supportive of building a BIPOC mental health workforce. Here, we present two programs currently in academic hospital settings that were created around the tenets of cultural and structural humility toward improving mental health outcomes in child and adolescent psychiatry.

APPLICATIONS
Cultural Humility Application: MGH - Center for Cross-Cultural Student Emotional Wellness - The Consortium Program

In 2018, the Massachusetts General Hospital Center for Cross-Cultural Student Emotional Wellness (MGH-CCCSEW) developed a year-long virtual program called the CCCSEW Consortium for secondary schools, colleges, and universities in the Boston, MA area. The program was a call to action from surrounding school faculty and administrators who noticed a concerning trend of Asian students exhibiting difficulties adjusting to campus and maladaptive coping behaviors. This was most palpable with the influx of Asian international students who were isolated from the larger student body, struggled with peer interpersonal relationships, and functioned below their academic potential.[11]

Conventional support offered was not effective when trying to address the mental health needs of Asian American and Asian international students. These students experienced marginalization in the realm of mental health given the stigma and lack of framework to contextualize their lived experience. The Consortium set out to help the schools recognize the unique needs of these students, their students' internal and external difficulties, and identify strategies to support them in a more productive way.

The Consortium program's goal was to create a virtual learning environment for educators from schools, initially within the New England region, though in recent years, it has expanded to outreach schools across the country. It offered participants clinical education on the mental health of Asian American and Asian international students as well as opportunities to interact and share their individual/institutional experiences through a peer-to-peer learning platform. Components of the Consortium included didactic teaching from clinicians well versed in cross-cultural mental health care, case presentation series, and subsequent live discussions. For schools/educators who benefited from a more individualized input, the Consortium offered specific case consultation. Structured to the academic year, the year-long program highlighted topics on cross-cultural approaches to specific mental health conditions such as depression, anxiety, impact of prejudice and discrimination on mental wellness, identity development in multi-cultural setting, intersectionality, parent–child/family relationship, cultural assimilation, and cultural perspectives on success.

An unspoken goal of the Consortium program is to instill and develop cultural humility for the participants, to avoid having schools and educators make overgeneralization of their students who are of Asian background, and for them to recognize the need for ongoing learning to support these students. During the 2020 - 2021 academic year, the emphasis on cultural humility intensified as the Consortium embarked on greater discussions and lectures for participants to learn the historic prejudice and discrimination of Asians in America, and help participants learn more about the impact of COVID-19 and anti-Asian racism on their students.

The CCCSEW Consortium strives for the member schools to take accountability on both an individual and institutional level in assessing their response and support to the Asian American and Asian international students. Through this interactive, dynamic process of cultural humility, Consortium participants commit to a learning process that is crucial in supporting the mental health of students.

Structural Humility Application: NYU DCAP Antiracism Task Force

Another example of institutional-level interventions that highlight social competence and related social humility is the antiracism task force (ARTF) developed by the New York University Department of Child and Adolescent Psychiatry. During Summer 2020, in the wake of the George Floyd murder and renewed interest in social justice issues, leaders in the department created an antiracism task force as a response to the moment.

The mission of the task force was to: (1) mobilize the department—faculty, staff, and trainees–to act to dismantle systemic racism in the department, institution, disciplines, and communities; (2) advocate for social justice; (3) empower and support BIPOC colleagues and patients; (4) encourage and support white members of the department to explore white privilege and its impact on systemic racism; and 5) develop and foster pathways to allyship.[12]

Structurally, the task force is composed of 5 pillars, each with distinct objectives to share the task force's unified mission:

1) Education and enrichment pillar:

Creating a speaker series of subject experts to help the department develop a shared framework for discussion and reflection regarding race, racism, and privilege.

2) Recruitment and retention pillar:

Creating a work environment that facilitates the hiring and retention of BIPOC faculty and trainees and provides mentorship for professional advancement.

3) Resource development and outreach:

Create a database of resources to facilitate learning and access to educational materials on race, racism, white privilege, intersectionality, allyship, and other related topics.

4) Practice and content review:

Address systemic racism and bias in the department's clinical and administrative content and processes (inward and outward facing).

5) Facilitated dialogues:

Conduct a series of small group discussions on issues of social identity on individual, institutional, and cultural levels. Dialogues create a safe space to lean into the discomfort of discussing race-related topics.

The ARTF has aspects that emphasize learning and change at both an individual and structural level. Invitations to the task force extend to all members of the department. The department chair also encourages participation in the program through protected time. These steps are meaningful when looking through a structural competence lens as they help to move the work beyond just the classic "physician-patient" interface into the larger departmental community, with the goal of departmental change leading to changes in the larger systems involved. As the task force includes all staff members, there are ample opportunities for exploring and challenging power dynamics that play out interpersonally and working toward increased humility.

The facilitated dialogues are small groups with 2 leaders, open to faculty, staff, and trainees of all backgrounds, and meet monthly to go through a curriculum on racial identity development and social justice. The dialogues featured sessions that challenge participants to explore their own social identities, experiences with privilege and racism, and microaggressions. Participants were encouraged to reflect on their experiences within the group and to take their experiences from the dialogue to influence their lives outside of work. In this way, the facilitated dialogues provided a space for culture humility and structural humility because all participants (both clinical and nonclinical) can play a role in affecting their own communities and finding space for advocacy, which is a larger goal of structural competence.[12]

The practices and content pillar provide an example of the structural competency aspects of "recognizing the structures that shape clinical interactions" and "developing an extra clinical language of structure."[7,13] In the first year of this pillar the initial goal was to conduct a literature review on racism and bias in clinical practice and developed recommendations on how to provide treatment, document patient care, and converse with colleagues and collaborators about patient racial/ethnic identification, experiences of racism/bias, and the impact of these experiences. This pillar recognizes that bias is often built right into the core everyday practices of our clinical work. Structural competency requires us to seek out and examine the "how" and "why" of our clinical practices and gain a better understanding of the societal upstream contributors of our current practices.[14]

Mezel positions structural humility as a component of structural competence that recognizes the limitations of the practice.[7,13] And these limitations are not an impediment but a reminder of the complexity of the issues and that the work is ongoing and we are a beginning of the conversation and not yet at an endpoint. The core features of cultural humility call for a lifelong commitment to self-evaluation and self-critique and not to be seen as obtaining a fixed set of knowledge.[5] While the NYU Anti-racism task force serves as an example of an approach to structural humility in an academic institution setting, the work is by nature imperfect and frequent reflection on the mission, processes, and impact on both the individual and structural level are an integral part of the group; in addition to an acceptance that, to achieve our stated goals, ongoing change and adaptation is essential.

CONCLUSION

Reducing disparities in mental health requires a concerted and collective approach that looks at the patient-clinician dyadic relationship, as well as the structural framework that trains the clinician and hosts that patient–clinician relationship. As the country moves toward an ever-increasing culturally diverse population, and a reckoning of the pervasiveness of systemic racism, the expectation for health care professionals to master competency in knowledge of a particular cultural group is insufficient and potentially harmful. Active appraisal of our awareness and continuous exploration and understanding of the lived experiences of others is the way forward in which clinicians can quantify what they know and don't know. Mental health professionals are positioned on the frontline in interfacing with youths and families distressed from the mental toll of systemic racism and discrimination, interpersonal acts of hate and rejection, and a lost sense of belonging. Cultural humility functions as a sustainable process of lifelong learning, promotes mental health care that is compassionate, and encourages engagement in advocacy for social justice causes on a systemic level. Collectively, these dynamic and ever-growing efforts will help assure that the mental health needs of BIPOC youths can be met, and a process of healing and overcoming can ensue to address mental health disparities.

CLINICS CARE POINTS

- When working with BIPOC youths, practicing cultural humility may entail discomfort in clinicians who may find themselves contending with their own biases and wrongdoings, and need to recover and repair trust with the patient.

- An Organization's commitment to supporting initiatives and training that promotes cultural humility is vital to positive outcomes.

- A clinician's capacity to explore and understand the lived experience of BIPOC youths facing racism and discrimination can provide healing and empowerment towards social justice.

DISCLOSURE

A.S. Li reports the following conflict of interest: chapter coauthor for Cultural Psychiatry in Children Adolescents and Families, American Psychiatric Publishing 2021. Q. Lang reports no financial relationships or interests. J. Cho reports the following conflict of interest: chapter coauthor for Cultural Psychiatry in Children Adolescents and Families, American Psychiatric Publishing 2021. V-S. Nguyen reports no financial relationships or interests. S. Nandakumar reports no financial relationships or interests.

REFERENCES

1. Institute of medicine (US) Committee on understanding and eliminating racial and ethnic disparities in health care. In: Smedley BD, Stith AY, Nelson AR, editors. Unequal treatment: Confronting racial and ethnic disparities in health care. Washington, DC: National Academies Press (US); 2003.
2. McGuire TG, Miranda J. New evidence regarding racial and ethnic disparities in mental health: policy implications. Health Aff (Millwood) 2008;27(2):393–403.
3. Center for Behavioral Health Statistics and Quality. Racial/ethnic differences in mental health service use among adults and adolescents (2015-2019) (Publication No. PEP21-07-01-002). Rockville, MD: Substance Abuse and Mental Health Services Administration. 2021. Available at: https://www.samhsa.gov/data/.
4. Hook J, Davis D, Owen J, et al. Cultural humility: measuring openness to culturally diverse clients. J Couns Psychol 2013;60:353–66.

5. Tervalon M, Murray-García J. Cultural humility versus cultural competence: a critical distinction in defining physician training outcomes in multicultural education. J Health Care Poor Underserved 1998;9(2):117–25.
6. Lekas HM, Pahl K, Lewis CF. Rethinking cultural competence: shifting to cultural humility health services insights 2020;13:1–4.
7. Metzl JM, Hansen H. Structural competency: theorizing a new medical engagement with stigma and inequality. Soc Sci Med 2014;103:126–33.
8. Hook J, Farrell J, Davis D, et al. Cultural humility and racial microaggression in counseling. J Couns Psychol 2016;63:269–77.
9. Duron J, Williams-Butler A, Schmidt A, et al. Mentors' experience of mentoring justice-involved adolescents: a narrative of developing cultural consciousness through connection. J Community Psychol 2020;48:2309–25.
10. Akerele O, McCall M, Aragam G. Healing ethno-racial trauma in Black communities: cultural humility as a driver of innovation. JAMA Psychiatry 2021;78:703–4.
11. Lim CT, Chen JA. A novel virtual partnership to promote Asian American and Asian international student mental health. Psychiatr Serv 2021;72:736–9.
12. NYU department of child and adolescent psychiatry anti-racism task force (ARTF) mission STatement. 2020. https://med.nyu.edu/departments-institutes/child-adolescent-psychiatry/about-us/anti-racism-task-force. Accessed October 30, 2021.
13. Metzl JM, Hansen H. Structural competency and psychiatry. JAMA Psychiatry 2018;75(2):115–6.
14. Hansen H, Braslow J, Rohrbaugh RM. From cultural to structural competency—training psychiatry residents to act on social determinants of health and institutional racism. JAMA Psychiatry 2018;75(2):117–8.

The Impact of Racism on the Health and Wellbeing of Black Indigenous and Other Youth of Color (BIPOC Youth)

Hasiya E. Yusuf, MBBS, MPH[a], Nikeea Copeland-Linder, PhD, MPH[b],
Andrea S. Young, PhD[c], Pamela A. Matson, PhD, MPH[a],
Maria Trent, MD, MPH[a],*

KEYWORDS

- Youth • Racism • Discrimination • Minorities • Minoritized
- Black, Indigenous And People of Color (BIPOC)

KEY POINTS

- Many minoritized (BIPOC) youth experience racial discrimination and victimization as early as the first decade of life.
- Racial discrimination in any form negatively impacts the health and wellbeing of BIPOC youth and may create barriers to accessing care.
- Parents convey various ethnic-racial socialization messages to their children, focused on instilling cultural pride, increasing the awareness of racial inequities, and providing strategies for coping with discrimination.
- Training and preparing health care providers to address racial trauma effectively and youth-targeted intervention programs can play important roles in mitigating the harmful effects of racism on the mental health of affected youth.

INTRODUCTION

The racial discrimination of minoritized populations (Latinos/Latinx/Hispanics, Asian/Pacific Islanders, Native Americans, Alaskan Natives, Black/African Americans, Middle Eastern Americans, and other ethnic and religious minorities) or Black, Indigenous, and People of Color (BIPOC) pervades nearly all facets of American society, negatively impacting various aspects of their lives.[1,2] BIPOC youth experience racism from a young age with increasing frequency as they age.[3] The impact of structural,

[a] Department of Pediatrics, Johns Hopkins University School of Medicine, Johns Hopkins University, 200 N Wolfe Street, Baltimore, MD 21287, USA; [b] Department of Psychiatry and Behavioral Sciences, Kennedy Krieger Institute, Johns Hopkins School of Medicine, 600 N Wolfe Street, Baltimore, MD 21205, USA; [c] Division of Child and Adolescent Psychiatry, Johns Hopkins School of Medicine, 1800 Orleans Street, Bloomberg 12 N, Baltimore, MD 21287 USA
* Corresponding authors.
E-mail addresses: hyusuf1@jhu.edu (H.E.Y.); mtrent2@jhmi.edu (M.T.)

Child Adolesc Psychiatric Clin N Am 31 (2022) 261–275
https://doi.org/10.1016/j.chc.2021.11.005
1056-4993/22/© 2021 Elsevier Inc. All rights reserved.

internalized, or interpersonal racism on the mental health and wellbeing of minoritized youth is well documented.[2,4] Both direct and vicarious racially motivated encounters (eg, racial discrimination of close family members or community) have adverse impacts on minoritized youth's health and wellbeing.[4,5] The goal of this article is to highlight the multiple ways in which racism affects the health of BIPOC youth, protective factors, and possible solutions.

RACISM AND YOUTH IN AMERICA

Racism is "a system of oppression that categorizes and stratifies social groups into 'races,' devalues and disadvantages those considered inferior, and differentially allocate to them valued societal resources and opportunities."[6] BIPOC youth are exposed to racial discrimination early in their lives, with many reporting racially motivated encounters during the first decade of life.[3] As an example, starting in preschool, schools label minoritized children difficult/disruptive and discipline them more often despite having similar behavior profiles to their peers. These experiences continue as they move through the education system and outside the classroom.[7,8] Many BIPOC youth have also had vicarious or direct encounters with the police by 7th grade.[9] U.S. population-based data finds BIPOC youth (across gender) have the highest personal encounters with law enforcement of any adolescent racial group in the United States (US), and BIPOC boys experience aggressive and intrusive treatments that are rare for white boys.[10] Substantial racial differences exist in police stops, with BIPOC youth more likely to be stopped by the police while driving.[10,11] It is noteworthy that frequent police contacts amplify adolescents' delinquent behaviors, ironically, what the correctional system seeks to combat.[11] This effect is further mediated by the psychological stress imposed by the experience.[12]

Involvement with the police exemplifies just one of the types of everyday experiences of racism for BIPOC youth. As reported by a recent study, BIPOC youth encounter up to 5 experiences of racial discrimination daily.[13] However, the worst racial provocations may result from structural racism. The force of institutional racism exerts its toll on BIPOC youths' access to resources, educational attainment, wealth accumulation, neighborhood structure, and other aspects of daily life[14–16] For example, socioeconomic and geographic divides have maintained a de facto state of segregation more than 6 decades after the Brown versus Board of education decision to desegregate U.S. schools.[17] Property taxes fund schools and the resultant impact of federal loan and housing policies in the U.S. segregated the US and have resulted in higher property values in white neighborhoods.[18] Consequently, better-funded schools in white communities offer better facilities, more expansive educational and extracurricular opportunities, and have more qualified teachers.[19,20] Conversely, schools in poor neighborhoods, which are disproportionately attended by minoritized populations, are often poorly equipped with dilapidated buildings, teachers who are stretched thin, and inadequate counseling staff.[19,21] These factors contribute to higher dropout rates, lower college attendance rates, and subsequently lower family incomes for BIPOC.[14,22] For BIPOC youth who successfully matriculate into college, similar roadblocks encountered in secondary school resurface. Minoritized youth often attend for-profit institutions, obtain certificates rather than bachelor's degrees, and major in fields with lower earning potentials than white students.[23] Income disparities persist even with educational achievement, especially for African Americans with college degrees who have just 75% of the wealth of white high school graduates.[14]

IMPACT OF RACISM ON HEALTH

All forms of racial discrimination, whether institutional, personally mediated, or internalized, negatively impact the health and wellbeing of BIPOC.[4] Historically, the inequitable distribution of health resources and other social determinants of health have created barriers to accessing care.[24,25] In addition, many BIPOC have a longstanding mistrust of the health care system, stemming from a long history of unethical experimentation on BIPOC people.[26,27] The shortage of BIPOC health care professionals, the history of segregated and differential treatment in health care, and more recently, the COVID-19 pandemic have worsened and unmasked the effect of this mistrust.[28,29] As an example, COVID-19 vaccination statistics reveal that BIPOC, who represent the population most affected by COVID-19 in terms of severity and fatality, have the highest vaccine hesitancy.[30] The structural racism that drives mistrust by BIPOC and the inequality it breeds extend beyond the pandemic to other aspects of the BIPOC experience. For instance, some researchers suggest that the disproportionate burden of obesity in BIPOC youth is rooted in structural racism - impacting black youth in particular.[31,32] Racism is associated with geographic segregation, and paired with lack of investment in these neighborhoods, leads to BIPOC living in "obesogenic environments" (food swamps, stores with ultraprocessed foods, high concentration of fast-food restaurants, and limited availability of healthy foods) - once again impacting black youth in particular.[31,33] Disparities also persist in the care of BIPOC youth. Implicit bias by providers and a misperception of a high threshold for pain by BIPOC patients results in poor pain management. BIPOC patients are significantly less likely to be prescribed opioid analgesics than their white counterparts with the same clinical condition.[34] Further, BIPOC patients presenting to the emergency department with bone fractures are less likely to be prescribed opioid analgesics and more likely not to receive any form of analgesia compared with white patients.[34,35]

Forces embedded in systemic racism also contribute to disparities in physical and mental health. BIPOC youth raised in low-income geographic milieus are more likely to use alcohol or marijuana.[36] Experiencing racism is associated with increased anxiety, depression, and overall mental health decline, with a similar but less pronounced influence on physical health.[37] Direct or indirect childhood exposure to racism is associated with poorer health outcomes and increased exposure to adversity that impacts health.[38] Many of these effects are far-reaching and not offset by higher levels of education or growing up in healthier environments.[37]

RACISM AND RISK BEHAVIORS

Research has shown that social rejection based on race impresses on behavior, including risk-taking.[39] Perception of racial discrimination leads to risky sexual behavior in BIPOC youth, and substance use facilitates this relationship.[40] The effect of social discrimination on sexual risk behavior is attenuated for BIPOC men with social support networks and structures. However, having a support system does not entirely mitigate the relationship between discrimination and risk behavior.[41] Racial discrimination indirectly impacts sexual risk behavior by triggering posttraumatic stress disorder (PTSD) in affected individuals.[42] Racially triggered PTSD, in turn, leads to heightened sexual risk-taking. Beyond sexual behavior, race-based discrimination may lead to aggressive behavior and substance abuse in adolescent and young adult BIPOC, particularly Black/African Americans.[43] Racial discrimination experienced at very young ages, well before any sexual activity, is associated with sexual behavior in later years.[44] For example, a group of minoritized sexually inactive children who experienced racial discrimination at young ages was found to engage in more sexual risk-taking behaviors 10 years later when they became sexually active compared with children of similar ages who did not report experiencing racial discrimination.[44]

DISPARITIES IN ACCESSING CARE

In its book, "*Unequal Treatment,*" the Institute of Medicine defined disparities in health care access as any difference in care not based on clinical needs or patients' treatment preferences.[45] Disparate access and receipt of health services in BIPOC have existed for centuries within the US. Despite years of effort to close the gaps in health care access for minoritized groups, they have persisted. Disparities in health care access for BIPOC exist on many levels. BIPOC youth are not only less likely to initiate treatment[46] but also less likely to stay in treatment[47] and receive adequate care.[48,49] Thus, even those youth and families who are able to overcome significant barriers to initiating services continue to experience barriers to remaining in treatment and/or receiving adequate care. Further, most minoritized youth have trouble receiving care from a consistent location. Unlike white families, many Black families receive care from emergency departments and community health centers, and Black children are less likely to be seen by a specialist compared with white children.[50] The causes of disparities in access to services are likely multifactorial and systemic. While stigma, treatment preferences, and understanding/knowledge of mental illness are often investigated as contributors to disparities in access to mental health services, these factors seem to explain only a small portion of the disparities.[51] Further, focusing on these factors may also overly pathologize medical mistrust in Black communities[52] and unduly place the burden of addressing disparate barriers to access on minoritized communities. Different treatment approaches-including engaging family members, culturally tailoring treatment, and increasing availability of mental health providers-may help reduce disparities in access to mental health care.[51] The ability of minoritized youth to access quality care is also affected by the geographic location of BIPOC, which do not often coincide with the distribution of health care facilities. Private, high-volume urban research-centered facilities known to provide better quality care are mainly situated closer to white residencies, creating a geographic barrier for minoritized populations.[24]

Research has demonstrated the broad impact of provider racial and ethnic bias on health disparities.[53] There is evidence of such bias influencing clinical decision-making.[53,54] Mental health treatment may be more susceptible to provider bias as decisions about treatment access, diagnosis, and disposition are often made by a single provider, compared with the team-based approaches now used in many other disciplines.[55] Of the psychology workforce, 5% are Hispanic or Latino/a, 0.3% American Indian or Alaska Native, 4% Asian, 4% Black, 1.5% multiracial, 84% non-Hispanic White, and 2% other racial/ethnic groups.[56] Representation among practicing psychiatrists is similar: 5.8% identify as Hispanic/Latino, 0.2% as American Indian, Alaska Native, Native Hawaiian, or Pacific Islander, 15.7% as Asian, 4.4% as Black, and 54.7% as white.[57]

On its part, the government has made efforts to improve access to care for BIPOC. Policies like the affordable care act (ACA) strive to improve access to care for young and underserved people and have successfully addressed some racial/ethnic disparities in health care access for BIPOC youth.[58] However, the determinants of health care access extend beyond ensuring insurance coverage for youth[39] and this approach may have shifted funds away from developmentally appropriate programs and services designed to meet the needs of gray area youth.

As an example, in a sample of youth with type 1 diabetes, BIPOC youth experienced the most barriers to accessing care, with many reporting frequent changes in care providers and roadblocks to scheduling appointments. As expected, these groups also experienced the most inconsistencies in glycemic control.[59] Similar barriers were encountered by minoritized 12th-grade high school students with autistic spectrum disorder (ASD) who have more unmet needs in receiving ASD care than white students.[60] For many BIPOC, challenges such as difficulty finding providers, scheduling health care visits, and finding specialties within the communities in which they reside also contribute significantly to limited care access.[50] BIPOC with neurologic conditions are 30% less likely to be seen by a neurology specialist in the outpatient department irrespective of age. Minoritized youth less than 35 years are 1.2x more likely than white youth of the same age to present with perforated appendicitis. This difference is thought to result from differences in socioeconomic status and access to needed care at this age.[61] Hence, being a BIPOC youth impacts the type, availability, and frequency of access to health care. BIPOC youth are unequivocally on the losing side of health care access.

ROLE OF GENERATIONAL TRAUMA AND DEPRIVATION ON HEALTH AND WELLBEING

In her 2005 book, Joy DeGruy introduced the concept of posttraumatic slave syndrome (PTSS), the intergenerational trauma created by a history of slavery and perpetuated by continued racial discrimination against African Americans.[62] Before the abolition of the slave trade, the practice of slavery brought untoward suffering and negatively impacted the health of African Americans. As enslaved people, African Americans endured years of maltreatment, malnourishment, poor health, and unfair separation from their families. Infants born to enslaved mothers were malnourished due to the limited time allowed for feeding by slave masters.[63] This translated to exceptionally high infant mortality rates whereby nearly a third of all infants born to enslaved parents died before their first year of life.[64] More than 150 years after the abolition of slavery, it has continued to have implications for African Americans in the present. A similar effect of generational trauma, known as "historical trauma symptoms," has been described for Native Americans.[65] According to DeGruy, the legacy of racial trauma frames behaviors and attitudes, and attitudes considered protective and necessary for survival in the slave era and carried forward through the years may undermine survival, health, and overall wellbeing today.[62] One example is the distrust of health care systems and providers borne out of a horrific history of unethical experimentation on BIPOC.[26] Some identified features of PTSS are a low sense of worth, the pervasive belief that one is inferior, and a propensity for aggressive behavior and persistent anger.[62] These behaviors breed anxiety, a sense of hopelessness, and risk for suicidal ideation and physical harm. It is theorized that involvement in gangs, poor relationships, and substance use are, on some level, the trickle-down effect of generational trauma.[66] The study seems to support the belief that generational trauma, present-day discrimination, and internalized racism morphs into attitudes, behaviors, and perceptions that, by extension, influence wellbeing and health outcomes. Findings from a systematic review on the vicarious effects of racism on health outcomes for children can be considered an allegory of the health impact of generational trauma of racism. In the study, vicarious racism was significantly associated with various health outcomes of children.[5] In the same vein, an amalgam of the historical footprint of slavery, racial segregation, ethnic subjugation, and past and ongoing discrimination continues to leave its negative mark on the health of BIPOC.

NAVIGATING WHITE SPACES AND EMOTIONAL STRESS

In "Black Faces, White Spaces," Carolyn Finney alludes to the differential access of whites and Blacks to American spaces and the prevalent framing of the environment as white.[67] From schools to residential areas, workplaces, public domains, and digital/virtual spaces, BIPOC youth have had to operate and thrive in spheres characterized as white spaces (spaces whereby BIPOC have limited numbers, aren't expected to be in, or are overlooked) as a matter of necessity and survival. Across these spaces, BIPOC tends to be in the statistical minority and need to adopt techniques to thrive or merely survive as the nondominant group. The reality of spatial distinctions by race is ingrained early in many BIPOC youths as families teach their children to abide by the construct of white dominance by instilling ideas of acceptable white space behaviors and code-switching (using one dialect or accent over another) to fit into white norms.[68] BIPOC youth are forced to confront negative stereotypes and pressured into behavior modifications that confirm the U.S.' pervasive but often unspoken categorization as a normatively white entity. They have had to compromise their true identities, prioritizing the comfort of white people to be accepted or tolerated in white spaces. Expectations to fit in or conform to white standards in such areas threaten their true identity and incite psychological, physical, and emotional stress. Black students who attend predominantly white schools face the nagging fear of being perceived as inferior and less intelligent by their white classmates and teachers, subtle and overt racial insensitivities, and pressures to prove their worth.[69,70] To divert racially motivated negative stereotypes, BIPOC students attempt to adapt through behavior modification (1 student recalls not asking questions in class to avoid being perceived as dumb) or change aspects of themselves to be viewed in a better light.[69] Minoritized youth face undue scrutiny and pressure to perform. Even among high achieving students in predominantly white schools, the racialization of achievement becomes a stressor as minoritized students question their capacities for academic feats leading them to doubt their aptitudes despite excelling at school. BIPOC who are not accustomed to the unspoken rules and expectations of white spaces risk being tokenized or slapped with subtly derogatory labels. Whether it is calling the police on a Black Yale student for napping in the common room, or the rising violence against Asian Americans in the COVID-19 pandemic, BIPOC youth in integrated but overwhelmingly white spaces have been surveilled, confronted, and affronted for engaging in activities that would be considered normal. Such persistent discrimination put BIPOC youth perpetually at a disadvantage and worsen racial disparities and health outcomes.[71]

CULTURALLY RELEVANT PROTECTIVE FACTORS FOR BIPOC YOUTH: ETHNIC-RACIAL SOCIALIZATION AND ETHNIC-RACIAL IDENTITY DEVELOPMENT.

Experiencing racism does not always result in maladaptive outcomes for youth. A growing body of research documents the protective role of cultural and familial factors that promote wellbeing among BIPOC in a society in which their ethnic or racial group is frequently devalued.[72,73] Some parenting strategies promote resilience in the context of racial stress.[74] Ethnic-racial socialization has been defined as a process by which parents or caregivers transmit messages to youth about race, ethnicity, and ethnic-racial dynamics.[73,75] This may include conveying explicit or implicit messages to youth about the value of their ethnic group or race and preparing them for the racism they may face. Ethnic-racial socialization has been associated with positive outcomes for youth, including behavioral competence, academic achievement, and reduced anxiety.[76–78]

Parents convey a variety of ethnic-racial socialization messages to their children. Research on ethnic-racial socialization has focused primarily on 4 types of messages.

Cultural socialization messages focus on instilling ethnic, racial, and cultural pride and teaching about cultural traditions. *Preparation for bias messages* focuses on increasing awareness of racial inequities and providing strategies for coping with prejudice and discrimination. *Promotion of mistrust* includes messages that emphasize the need for caution and wariness about other groups. The use of this strategy does not involve providing strategies for coping. *Egalitarian messages* deemphasize ethnic and racial group membership and place value on individual characteristics needed to succeed in the dominant culture.[73] The bulk of empirical studies has focused on *cultural socialization* and *preparation for bias messages*. According to the seminal review conducted by Hughes, the percent of Black parents who report conveying cultural socialization messages ranges from 33% to 80%, and 67% to 90% report using preparation for bias messages.[73] Several factors influence the frequency and type of messages that parents transmit to youth, including the child's age, gender, neighborhood context, the nature of discriminatory experiences as well as parental characteristics.[79,80] In general, studies suggest that parents tend to engage in more frequent racial socialization during adolescence.[81] The content of messages may vary as a function of the developmental stage. Research indicates that parents report conveying more cultural socialization messages to younger children and more preparation for bias messages to older youth.[81]

Specific types of ethnic-racial socialization messages vary in how they relate to youth outcomes, particularly in the context of discriminatory experiences. Studies indicate that *cultural socialization* messages that emphasize instilling racial pride mitigate the harmful effects of racial discrimination on psychological wellbeing, including anxiety, anger, and delinquency.[76,78,82] Studies of the protective role of *preparation of bias* messages have found that these messages attenuated the effects of discrimination on delinquency and decreased the impact of discrimination on perceived stress.[82,83] Some research suggests that *promotion of mistrust* is associated with poorer psychological outcomes.[74] However, the protective role of specific types of ethnic racial socialization messages may vary for different ethnic groups. For example, in a study of Asian American youth, *promotion of mistrust* and *cultural socialization* messages were protective for U.S.-born Filipino youth, but for Korean American youth, *preparation of bias* messages reduced depressive symptoms for youth experiencing discrimination.[84] Although racial socialization has been conceptualized as a process that occurs between parents and children, as youth move through adolescence, they receive racial socialization messages from adults and peers in many contexts, including schools, churches, and the media.

Parents also use ethnic-racial socialization messages to promote positive ethnic-racial identity, a pivotal aspect of self-worth for many youths that has been associated with healthy psychological functioning and goal-oriented behavior, and problem-solving coping.[85,86] Identity development is a complex process through which individuals develop a sense of self within a particular group, culture, or ethnicity.[87] Identity formation is an essential task of adolescence that can impact present and future relationships, self-perception, physical, mental, and emotional wellbeing.[87] For Black youth, racial identity exploration and attunement with their culture and heritage is vital to developing a healthy sense of self and communal belonging. The centrality of race to identity shapes racial identity development and is acquired mainly through adult influences. Youth with well-developed sense of ethnic-racial identity have higher private regard (individuals' personal feelings and assessment of their race) and enjoy "racial centrality" (an individual's emphasis of their membership of a racial group in defining themselves).[88] A strong ethnic-racial identity in Black youth can offset the impact of racial discrimination at school.[89] In fact, certain scholars have gone a step further to suggest that the education of Black youth be optimized to include Black history from a positive lens. Proponents argue that by highlighting their ancestors' strengths, capabilities, and accomplishments in the face of untoward hardship, the psychological barriers encountered by Black students will be minimized.[90] High levels of centrality and private regard were shown to offset the depressive effect of racial discrimination in Black adolescents.[91]

Other schools of thought posit that the processes involved in ethnic-racial identity development can have both benefits and pitfalls. On the one hand, exposure of Black youth to information about their cultures promotes racial centrality, a measure of racial identity development.[92] Ethnic-racial socialization communications that emphasize ethnic and racial pride and history positively impact ethnic-racial identity development.[55] On the other hand, racial centrality, a proxy of racial identity, leads to public regard (one's perception of how others view their race), and Black youth who define themselves by their racial identities may be more sensitive to such perceptions.[93,94] Perception of discrimination in students can demotivate them from striving academically due to feelings of lower self-perceived competence.[95] Nonetheless, the upside of acculturation and promoting ethnic-racial identity development is not lost on parents, particularly mothers of Black youth who racially socialize their children from a young age, many from as early as the fifth grade.[55,95]

PROMISING APPROACHES TO FACILITATE THRIVING/PATHWAYS TO RECOVERY

As the causes of racial and ethnic disparities in health are multifactorial, the solutions should be multifaceted. Health care providers, therapists, and community interventionists may benefit from training that prepares them to effectively address racial trauma experienced by the youth and families they serve. Prevention and intervention programs for BIPOC should incorporate strengths-based approaches that capitalize on the resilience and rich legacy of racial socialization among BIPOC families. For example, the Strong African American Families Project (SAAF), an empirically validated preventive intervention program designed to avert risk-taking behaviors in youth, incorporates ethnic-racial socialization into the curriculum.[96] Engaging, Managing, and Bonding through Race (EMBRace) is a clinical intervention that uses racial socialization to address racial stress and trauma and promote adaptive coping in BIPOC families.[97]

The lay health worker (LHW) model of care is another promising solution.[98] LHWs are typically nonprofessional providers who are members of the communities that they serve. LHWs have been used in several contexts/roles. LHWs as liaisons or patient and family navigators help facilitate access and orient families to complex systems of care. Auxiliary care models use LHWs to help provide psychoeducation, identify treatment barriers, and provide phone call reminders for appointments and other tasks. In a third model, task-sharing, LHWs deliver evidence-based practices as part of a team or as the primary providers. Results from research studies of the efficacy of LHW for youth with mental health concerns in the US have been limited but promising.[98]

In closing, BIPOC youth face challenges to healthy development associated with their racial-ethnic and cultural identities in the U.S. Attacks on the community and failure to acknowledge and rectify the history of trauma or embracing differences as normative in spaces where children live (eg, education), and the continued receipt of differential treatment where they shouldn't (eg, justice systems) continues to undermine wellbeing. This leaves the responsibility for protecting the psyche and developmental trajectories for BIPOC children and adolescents largely to their BIPOC parents, families, and communities without substantial societal accountability. Efforts to shift the US to a postracial society have been thwarted by the rise in hate groups and unaddressed manifestations of the longstanding generational trauma and depriva-tion,[62] such that even families with higher educational attainment and socioeconomic status find themselves explaining to their children and adolescents that they belong to a "caste" and how to protect themselves as they increasingly navigate the world without them.[99,100] While professional health organizations have embraced disman-tling racism or its effects in clinical service as an important challenge worth tack-ling,[101,102] tremendous investments to shift the narrative on the racial value both inside and outside of health care will be critical for preventing adversity and achieving health equity for BIPOC children, youth, and families.

CONFLICT OF INTEREST STATEMENT

Dr. Trent receives funding from the National Institutes of Health (NINR, NICHD, and NIMHD) and research supplies from SpeeDx, LLC through Johns Hopkins University. She also serves on the Trojan Sexual Health Advisory Council (Church and Dwight, Inc.). Dr. Young has received/receives research support from NIDA, Brain & Behavior Research Foundation (BBRF), Supernus Pharmaceuticals, and Psychnostics, LLC. She has served as a consultant to NIH, PCORI, and the University of Montana's Amer-ican Indian/Alaska Native Clinical & Translational Research Program and on the Board of Directors for Helping Give Away Psychological Science and is on the editorial board for the Journal of Clinical Child and Adolescent Psychology and Evidence-Based Practice in Child and Adolescent Mental Health.

REFERENCES

1. Cohen A, Ekwueme PO, Sacotte KA, et al. "Melanincholy": a Qualitative explo-ration of youth media Use, vicarious racism, and perceptions of health. J Adolesc Health 2021;69(2):288–93.

2. Kalin NH. Impacts of structural racism, socioeconomic deprivation, and Stigma-tization on mental health. Am J Psychiatry 2021;178(7):575–8.

3. Nagata JM, Ganson KT, Sajjad OM, et al. Prevalence of perceived racism and discrimination among US children aged 10 and 11 Years: the adolescent Brain Cognitive development (ABCD) study. JAMA Pediatr 2021;175(8):861–3.

4. Trent M, Dooley DG, Dougé J, et al. The impact of racism on child and adoles-cent health. Pediatrics 2019;144(2). https://doi.org/10.1542/peds.2019-1765.

5. Heard-Garris NJ, Cale M, Camaj L, et al. Transmitting Trauma: a systematic re-view of vicarious racism and child health. Soc Sci Med 2018;199:230–40.

6. Priest N, Doery K, Truong M, et al. Updated systematic review and meta-analysis of studies examining the relationship between reported racism and health and well-being for children and youth: a Protocol. BMJ open. Available at: https://bmjopen.bmj.com/content/11/6/e043722.abstract. Accessed September 29, 2021.

7. Gilliam WD, Maupin AN, Reyes CR, et al. Do early Educators' implicit Biases regarding sex and race relate to behavior expectations and Recommendations of preschool Expulsions and suspensions?. 2016. Available at:https://www.semanticscholar.org/paper/Do-Early-Educators%E2%80%99-Implicit-Biases-Regarding-Sex-Gilliam-Ph./95eb66c67cd968551df29f7e374c1a253bd6b8ce. . Accessed October 5, 2021.

8. Huang FL. Do Black students misbehave more? Investigating the differential involvement hypothesis and out-of-school suspensions. J Educ Res 2018; 111(3):284–94.

9. Shedd C unequal City: race, schools, and perceptions of Injustice. Russell Sage Foundation; 2015. Available at: http://www.jstor.org/stable/10.7758/978161 0448529.

10. Geller A. Youth–police contact: Burdens and inequities in an adverse childhood experience. AJPH 2014–2017;121:111, 1300_1308.

11. Slocum LA, Ann Wiley S, Esbensen F-A. The importance of being Satisfied: a Longitudinal exploration of police contact, Procedural Injustice, and subsequent delinquency. Criminal Justice Behav 2016;43(1):7–26.

12. Del Toro J, Lloyd T, Buchanan SK, et al. The criminogenic and psychological effects of police stops on adolescent black and Latino boys. Proc Natl Acad Sci Apr 2019;116(17):8261–8.

13. English D, Lambert SF, Tynes BM, et al. Daily multidimensional racial discrimination among Black U.S. American adolescents. J Appl Dev Psychol 2020;66: 101068.

14. Statista. U.S educational attainment, by ethnicity. 2018. Available at: https://www. statista.com/statistics/184264/educational-attainment-by-enthnicity/. Accessed October 2, 2021.

15. Barkan SE, Rocque M. Socioeconomic status and racism as Fundamental causes of Street Criminality. Crit Crim 2018;26(2):211–31.

16. Castro-Ramirez F, Al-Suwaidi M, Garcia P, et al. Racism and Poverty are barriers to the treatment of youth mental health concerns. J Clin Child Adolesc Psychol 2021;0(0):1–13.

17. Orfield G, Ee J, Frankenberg E, et al. Brown at 62: school segregation by race, poverty, and state. Los Angeles, CA: the Civil Rights Project-Proyecto Derechos Civiles at UCLA. 2016. Available at: https://eric.ed.gov/?id=ED565900. Accessed October 6, 2021.

18. Economic Policy Institute. The color of law: a Forgotten history of how Our government segregated America. Available at: https://www.epi.org/publication/the-color-of-law-a-forgotten-history-of-how-our-government-segregated-america/. Accessed October 24, 2021.

19. Gamoran A, An BP. Effects of school segregation and school resources in a changing policy context. Educ Eval Policy Anal 2016;38(1):43–64.

20. Miller J, Garran AM. The web of institutional racism. Smith Coll Stud Social Work 2007;77(1):33–67.

21. García E. Schools are still segregated, and black children are paying a price. Economic policy Institute. 2020. Available at: https://eric.ed.gov/?id=ED603475. Accessed October 6, 2021.

22. Median Statista. Household income by race or ethnic group. 2019. Available at: https://www.statista.com/statistics/233324/median-household-income-in-the-united-states-by-race-or-ethnic-group/. Accessed October 2, 2021.

23. Libassi CJ. The Neglected college race gap: racial disparities among college completers. 2018. Center for American progress. 2018. Available at: https://www. americanprogress.org/issues/education-postsecondary/reports/2018/05/23/4511 86/neglected-college-race-gap-racial-disparities-among-college-completers/. Accessed October 6, 2021.

24. Institute of Medicine (U.S. Committee on understanding and Eliminating racial and ethnic disparities in health care. In: Smedley BD, Stith AY, Nelson AR, editors. Unequal treatment: Confronting racial and ethnic disparities in health care. Washington (D.C.): National Academies Press (U.S.); 2003. 3, Assessing Potential Sources of Racial and Ethnic Disparities in Care: Patient- and System-Level Factors. Available from: https://www.ncbi.nlm.nih.gov/books/NBK220359/.

25. Garney W, Wilson K, Ajayi KV, et al. Social-ecological barriers to access to healthcare for adolescents: a Scoping review. Int J Environ Res Public Health 2021;18(8):4138.

26. Spigner C. Medical apartheid: the dark history of medical experimentation on black Americans from colonial times to the present. J Natl Med Assoc 2007; 99(9):1074–5.

27. Rodriguez MA, García R. First, do No harm: the U.S. Sexually transmitted disease experiments in Guatemala. Am J Public Health 2013;103(12):2122–6.

28. Feagin J, Bennefield Z. Systemic racism, and U.S. health care. Soc Sci Med 2014;103:7–14.

29. Baptiste DL, Commodore-Mensah Y, Alexander KA, et al. Shedding light on racial and health inequities in the USA. J Clin Nurs 2020;29(15-16):2734–6.

30. Reverby SM. Racism, disease, and vaccine refusal: people of color are dying for access to COVID-19 vaccines. PLOS Biol 2021;19(3):e3001167.

31. Aaron DG, Stanford FC. Is obesity a manifestation of systemic racism? A ten-point strategy for study and intervention. J Intern Med 2021;290(2):416–20.

32. Mwendwa DT, Gholson G, Sims RC, et al. Coping with perceived racism: a significant factor in the development of obesity in African American Women? J Natl Med Assoc 2011;103(7):602–8.

33. Mackey ER, Burton ET, Cadieux A, et al. Addressing structural racism is critical for Ameliorating the childhood obesity Epidemic in black youth. Child Obes 2021. https://doi.org/10.1089/chi.2021.0153.

34. Ghoshal M, Shapiro H, Todd K, et al. Chronic Noncancer pain management and systemic racism: time to move toward equal care standards. J Pain Res 2020; 13:2825–36.

35. Todd KH, Deaton C, D'Adamo AP, et al. Ethnicity, and analgesic practice. Ann Emerg Med 2000;35(1):11–6.

36. Currier D, Patton G, Sanci L, et al. Socioeconomic disadvantage, mental health and substance Use in young men in emerging adulthood. Behav Med 2021; 47(1):31–9.

37. Paradies Y, Ben J, Denson N, et al. Racism as a determinant of health: a systematic review and meta-analysis. PLOS ONE 2015;10(9):e0138511.

38. Priest N, Paradies Y, Trenerry B, et al. A systematic review of studies examining the relationship between reported racism and health and wellbeing for children and young people. Soc Sci Med 2013;95:115–27.

39. Jamieson JP, Koslov K, Nock MK, et al. Experiencing discrimination Increases risk taking. Psychol Sci 2013;24(2):131–9.

40. Stock ML, Gibbons FX, Peterson LM, et al. The effects of racial discrimination on the HIV-risk cognitions and behaviors of Black adolescents and young adults. Health Psychol 2013;32(5):543–50. https://doi.org/10.1037/a0028815.

41. Bowleg L, Burkholder GJ, Massie JS, et al. Racial discrimination, social support, and sexual HIV risk among Black heterosexual men. AIDS Behav 2013;17(1): 407–18.

42. Bowleg L, Fitz CC, Burkholder GJ, et al. Racial discrimination, and posttraumatic stress symptoms as pathways to sexual HIV risk behaviors among urban Black heterosexual men. AIDS Care 2014;26(8):1050–7.

43. Xie TH, Ahuja M, McCutcheon VV, et al. Associations between racial and socioeconomic discrimination and risk behaviors among African-American adolescents and young adults: a latent class analysis. Soc Psychiatry Psychiatr Epidemiol 2020;55:1479–89. https://doi.org/10.1007/s00127-020-01884-y.

44. Roberts ME, Gibbons FX, Gerrard M, et al. From racial discrimination to risky sex: Prospective relations involving peers and parents. Dev Psychol 2012; 48(1):89–102.

45. Institute of Medicine (U.S.) Committee on understanding and Eliminating Racial and Ethnic Disparities in Health Care. In: Smedley BD, Stith AY, Nelson AR, editors. . Unequal treatment: Confronting Racial and ethnic Disparities in health care. Washington, DC: National Academies Press (U.S.); 2003. p. 29–79. Available at: http://www.ncbi.nlm.nih.gov/books/NBK220358/. Accessed October 4, 2021.

46. Merikangas KR, He J, Burstein M, et al. Service utilization for lifetime mental disorders in U.S. adolescents: results of the National Comorbidity Survey-Adolescent Supplement (NCS-A). J Am Acad Child Adolesc Psychiatry 2011; 50(1):32–45.

47. Young AS, Horwitz SM, Findling RL, et al. Parents' perceived treatment match and treatment retention over 12 months among youth in the LAMS study. Psychiatr Serv 2016;67(3):310–5.

48. Saloner B, Carson N, Cook BL. Episodes of mental health treatment among a nationally representative sample of children and adolescents. Med Care Res Rev 2014;71(3):261–79.

49. Fontanella CA, Hiance-Steelesmith DL, Gilchrist R, et al. Quality of care for Medicaid-enrolled youth with bipolar disorders. Adm Policy Ment Health 2015; 42(2):126–38.

50. Gallarde-Kim S, Smith C, Roy Shreya. Health care needs, access to care, and experiences of racism for black children and youth with special health care needs and their families. OCCYSHN. 2020. Available at: https://www.ohsu.edu/sites/default/files/2020-10/OCCYSHN%202020%20NA%20Ch.3.pdf. Accessed October 8, 2021.

51. Cook BL, Hou SS-Y, Lee-Tauler SY, et al. A review of mental health and mental health care disparities research: 2011-2014. Med Care Res Rev 2019;76(6): 683–710.

52. Buchanan NT, Wiklund LO. Why clinical science must change or die: integrating intersectionality and social justice. Women Ther 2020;43(3–4):309–29.

53. Chapman EN, Kaatz A, Carnes M. Physicians, and implicit bias: how doctors may unwittingly perpetuate health care disparities. J Gen Intern Med 2013; 28(11):1504–10.

54. Merino Y, Adams L, Hall WJ. Implicit bias and mental health professionals: priorities and directions for research. Psychiatr Serv 2018;69(6):723–5.

55. Peck SC, Brodish AB, Malanchuk O, et al. Racial/ethnic socialization and identity development in Black families: the role of parent and youth reports. Dev Psychol 2014;50(7):1897–909. https://doi.org/10.1037/a0036800.

56. Lin L, Stamm K, Christidis P. Demographics of the U.S. Psychology workforce: Findings from the 2007-16 American community Survey: (506742018-001). Published online 2018. doi:10.1037/e506742018-001

57. Wyse R, Hwang W-T, Ahmed AA, et al. Diversity by race, ethnicity, and sex within the U.S. Psychiatry Physician workforce. Acad Psychiatry 2020;44(5): 523–30.

58. Lipton BJ, Decker SL, Sommers BD. The affordable care act appears to have Narrowed racial and ethnic disparities in insurance coverage and access to care among young adults. Med Care Res Rev 2019;76(1):32–55.

59. Valenzuela JM, Seid M, Waitzfelder B, et al. Prevalence of and disparities in barriers to care experienced by youth with type 1 diabetes. J Pediatr 2014;164(6): 1369–75.e1.

60. Taylor JL, Henninger NA. Frequency and correlates of service access among youth with autism transitioning to adulthood. J Autism Dev Disord 2015;45(1): 179–91.

61. Zogg CK, Scott JW, Jiang W, et al. Differential access to care: the role of age, insurance, and income on race/ethnicity-related disparities in adult perforated appendix admission rates. Surgery 2016;160(5):1145–54.

62. DeGruy LJ. Post Traumatic slave syndrome: America's legacy of enduring Injury and healing. Milwaukie(Oregon): Uptone Press; 2005.

63. Green VL, Killings NL, Clare CA. The historical, psychosocial, and cultural context of Breastfeeding in the African American community. Breastfeed Med 2021;16(2):116–20.

64. Steckel RH. A Dreadful childhood: the excess mortality of American slaves. Soc Sci Hist 1986;10(4):427–65.

65. The Professional Counselor. Examining the theory of historical trauma among native Americans. Available at: https://tpcjournal.nbcc.org/examining-the-theory-of-historical-trauma-among-native-americans/. Accessed October 22, 2021.

66. Ford BJ. Transmission of generational trauma in African American gang members. Available at: https://www.proquest.com/docview/1501633434/abstract/DC7FDB6507A44123PQ/1. Accessed October 4, 2021.

67. Finney C. Black faces, white spaces: Reimagining the relationship of African Americans to the Great Outdoors. UNC Press Books; 2014. Available at: https://uncpress.org/book/9781469614489/black-faces-white-spaces/. Accessed on October 6, 2021.

68. Ragland K. Black Skin in white spaces. Women, Gend Families Color 2020;8(2): 141–6. https://doi.org/10.5406/womgenfamcol.8.2.0141.

69. Griffith AN, Hurd NM, Hussain SB. I didn't come to school for this": a qualitative examination of experiences with race-related stressors and coping Responses among black students attending a predominantly white institution. J Adolesc Res 2019;34(2):115–39.

70. Linley JL. Racism here, racism there, racism everywhere: the racial realities of minoritized peer socialization agents at a historically white institution. J Coll Student Development 2018;59(1):21–36.

71. Anderson E. The white space." Sociology of race and ethnicity 2015;1(1):10–21.

72. Berkel C, Murry VM, Hurt TR, et al. It takes a village: protecting rural African American youth in the context of racism. J Youth Adolesc 2009;38(2):175–88.

73. Hughes D, Rodriguez J, Smith EP, et al. Parents' ethnic-racial socialization practices: a review of research and directions for future study. Dev Psychol 2006; 42(5):747–70.

74. Varner FA, Hou Y, Hodzic T, et al. Racial discrimination experiences and African American youth adjustment: the role of parenting profiles based on racial socialization and involved-vigilant parenting. Cultur Divers Ethnic Minor Psychol 2018; 24(2):173–86.

75. Lesane-Brown CL. A review of race socialization within Black families. Dev Rev 2006;26(4):400–26.

76. Bannon WM, McKay MM, Chacko A, et al. Cultural pride reinforcement as a dimension of racial socialization protective of urban African American child anxiety. Families Soc 2009;90(1):79–86.

77. Caughy MO, O'Campo PJ, Randolph SM, et al. The influence of racial socialization practices on the Cognitive and behavioral competence of African American Preschoolers. Child Development 2002;73(5):1611–25.

78. Wang M-T, Henry DA, Smith LV, et al. Parental ethnic-racial socialization practices and children of color's psychosocial and behavioral adjustment: a systematic review and meta-analysis. Am Psychol 2020;75(1):1–22.

79. Saleem FT, English D, Busby DR, et al. The impact of African American parents' racial discrimination experiences and perceived neighborhood cohesion on their racial socialization practices. J Youth Adolesc 2016;45(7):1338–49.

80. Saleem FT, Lambert SF, Stock ML, et al. Examining changes in African American mothers' racial socialization patterns during adolescence: racial discrimination as a predictor. Dev Psychol 2020;56(8):1610–22.

81. McHale SM, Crouter AC, Kim J-Y, et al. Mothers' and Fathers' racial socialization in African American families: implications for youth. Child Development 2006; 77(5):1387–402.

82. Dotterer AM, James A. Can parenting microprotections buffer against adolescents' experiences of racial discrimination? J Youth Adolesc 2018;47(1):38–50.

83. Burt CH, Simons RL. Interpersonal racial discrimination, ethnic-racial socialization, and offending: risk and resilience among African American Females. Justice Q 2015;32(3):532–70.

84. Park M, Choi Y, Yasui M, et al. Racial discrimination and the moderating effects of racial and ethnic socialization on the mental health of Asian American youth. Child Development 2021. https://doi.org/10.1111/cdev.13638.

85. Brody GH, Kim S, Murry VM, et al. Protective longitudinal paths linking child competence to behavioral problems among African American Siblings. Child Development 2004;75(2):455–67.

86. McBride Murry V, Brody GH, McNair LD, et al. Parental involvement promotes rural African American youths' self-pride and sexual self-Concepts. J Marriage Fam 2005;67(3):627–42.

87. Ragelienė T. Links of adolescents identity development and relationship with peers: a systematic literature review. J Can Acad Child Adolesc Psychiatry 2016;25(2):97–105.

88. Yip T. Ethnic identity in everyday life: the influence of identity development status. Child Dev 2014;85(1):205–19.

89. Leath S, Mathews C, Harrison A, et al. Racial identity, racial discrimination, and classroom engagement outcomes among black Girls and boys in predominantly black and predominantly white school districts. Am Educ Res J 2019;56(4): 1318–52.

90. Gray DL, Hope EC, Matthews JS. Black and belonging at school: a case for interpersonal, instructional, and institutional opportunity structures. null 2018; 53(2):97–113.

91. Seaton EK, Iida M. Racial discrimination, and racial identity: daily moderation among Black youth. Am Psychol 2019;74(1):117–27.

92. Sullivan JM, Platenburg GN. From black-ish to blackness: an analysis of black information sources' influence on black identity development. J Black Stud 2017;48(3):215–34.

93. Nioplias A, Chapman-Hilliard C, Jones BJ. Minority status stress, racial centrality, and racial socialization as predictors of Black Americans' preference for counselor race in a United States sample. Counselling Psychol Q 2018;31(4): 428–45.

94. Hudgens TM, Kurtz-Costes B, Swinton A, et al. Race centrality and racial socialization in African American adolescents: gender differences in identity development. 2007. Available at: http://bkcostes.web.unc.edu/files/2013/11/Hudgens-et-al-sra-08.pdf. Accessed October 4, 2021.

95. Tang S, McLoyd VC, Hallman SK. Racial socialization, racial identity, and academic attitudes among African American adolescents: examining the moderating influence of parent–adolescent communication. J Youth Adolesc 2016; 45(6):1141–55.

96. Brody GH, Kogan SM, Chen Y, et al. Long-term effects of the strong African American families program on youths' conduct problems. J Adolesc Health 2008;43(5):474–81.

97. Anderson RE, McKenny M, Mitchell A, et al. EMBRacing racial stress and trauma: preliminary feasibility and coping responses of a racial socialization intervention. J Black Psychol 2018;44(1):25–46.

98. Barnett ML, Luis Sanchez BE, Green Rosas Y, et al. Future directions in lay health worker involvement in children's mental health services in the U.S. J Clin Child Adolesc Psychol 2021;0(0):1–13.

99. Gross T. It's more than racism: Isabel Wilkerson explains America's "caste" system. NPR. 2020. Available at: https://www.npr.org/2020/08/04/898574852/its-more-than-racism-isabel-wilkerson-explains-america-s-caste-system. Accessed October 24, 2021.

100. Wilkerson I. Caste (Oprah's Book Club): the Origins of Our Discontents. Reprint edition. Random House; New York: 2020.

101. Svetaz MV, Barral R, Kelley MA, et al. Inaction is not an option: using Antiracism approaches to address health inequities and racism and Respond to current challenges affecting youth. J Adolesc Health 2020;67(3):323–5.

102. Society for Adolescent Health. Anti-racism Toolkit. Available at: https://www.adolescenthealth.org/Resources/Anti-Racism-Toolkit.asp. Accessed October 22, 2021.

Nurturing Children's Mental Health Body and Soul

Confronting American Child Psychiatry's Racist Past to Reimagine Its Antiracist Future

Rupinder K. Legha, MD, PC[a],*, Angélica Clayton, BA[b],
Lindsay Yuen, BA[c], Kimberly Gordon-Achebe, MD[d]

KEYWORDS

- Antiracism • Racism • White supremacy • Child mental health • History of medicine

KEY POINTS

- The history of American child psychiatry reveals its legacy of racism and white supremacy, particularly its refusals of white supremacy.
- Child psychiatry has neglected and even perpetuated the intergenerational trauma suffered by minoritized children and families.
- By refusing to confront racial injustice, it has centered on white children's protection and overlooked their role in white supremacist violence.
- An antiracist present and future for the profession demands a profound historical reckoning and comprehensive reimagining.
- Asking better questions using bold and radical frameworks, like Critical Race Theory and abolition, advances antiracism in child psychiatry more than seeking reductive answers using established frameworks, like health disparities.

INTRODUCTION
Child Psychiatry's Response to Jacob Blake's Shooting

August 2020. Three young brothers watch as police officers shoot their father, paralyzing him from the back down. The American Academy of Child and Adolescent Psychiatrists (AACAP) issues a statement condemning "the actions of a few officers," while supporting the majority who "serve with honor and professionalism." Noting the shooting "represent[s] a failure to... protect and serve," it recommends "[e]ffective screening and training of police officers with mandated antiracist and implicit bias

[a] 4859 West Slauson Avenue, #693, Los Angeles, CA 90056, USA; [b] Program in the History of Medicine and Science, Yale University, 320 York Street, New Haven, CT 06511, USA; [c] University of California Irvine School of Medicine, 1001 Health Sciences Road, Irvine, CA 92617, USA; [d] Department of Psychiatry, Division of Child and Adolescent Psychiatry, University of Maryland School of Medicine, 701 West Pratt Street, 4th Floor, Baltimore, MD 21201, USA
* Corresponding author.
E-mail address: antiracistmd@gmail.com

Child Adolesc Psychiatric Clin N Am 31 (2022) 277–294
https://doi.org/10.1016/j.chc.2021.11.006
1056-4993/22/© 2021 Elsevier Inc. All rights reserved.

training.…. ." AACAP asserts its "mission to promote the healthy development of children, adolescents, and families through advocacy, education, and research" and its "resolute support for the principle that Black Lives Matter" (BLM).[1]

August 2020. Two months have passed as 500,000 people joined BLM protests in the streets, demanding defunding the police.[2] *Abolition* aims to dismantle the *prison industrial complex*, the *carceral logic* prioritizing punishment to solve everyday problems, and the *carceral state*'s reach in education, social services, and health care.[3] Movement for Black Lives (M4BL) policy platforms reject AACAP's few bad apples contention, denying the plausibility of reforming or training an institution, birthed in slavery and criminalizing nonwhite bodies by design. *Abolition medicine* echoes the M4BL agenda, calling for historical redress through *reparations* and transforming the upstream structures, like policing, enabling the downstream violence devastating the lives of Jacob Blake and his children.[4] Within this context, the AACAP statement seems anachronistic.

August 2020. Nearly 70 years have passed as AACAP formed and Emmett Till was lynched, advancing a centuries-long arc of white supremacist state violence. Families were ripped apart during slavery; parents lynched during Jim Crow, their children forced into chain gangs; teenagers shot for wearing a hooded sweatshirt or whistling. The *intergenerational trauma* wrought by slavery and *settler colonialism* is immeasurable. The January 6th Capitol building storming captures how the *white rage* driving these genocidal campaigns persists.[5] But AACAP fails to reference these historical arcs or to mandate public health initiatives challenging this state violence and the racism fueling it. The message white children internalize witnessing a white police officer brutalizing a Black family and subsequently exonerated for it goes unchecked. AACAP's support for BLM is contradicted by its lack of antiracist orientation, which instead suggests a racist one.[6]

Serving Children's Mental Health Body and Soul: Confronting a Racist Past to Reimagine an Antiracist Future

AACAP's statement opens a window into American child psychiatry's legacy of racism and *white supremacy*, which this paper unpacks, connects to current inequities, and disrupts by reimagining an *antiracist* future. Alondra Nelson's history of the Black Panther Party's (BPP) health activism inspires the title, borrowed from a 1972 BPP's conference, whereby a banner proclaimed: "Serve the people body and soul."[7] Nurturing *all* children's mental health body and soul, this paper rejects reductive answers provided by existing frameworks and invites new questions inspired by bolder ones, like *abolition*, *decolonization*, and *Critical Race Theory* (CRT) (**Box 1**). Introducing sections with questions implicates readers in remaking this history into an *antiracist* future. Probing history demonstrates how child psychiatry has neglected the *intergenerational trauma* suffered by minoritized children and families and even perpetuated it. Its refusal to link child mental health to the legacies of slavery and *settler colonialism* upholds *white supremacy* while impeding antiracist change. **Box 1** features conceptual frameworks; **Box 2** provides key definitions (bolded); and images humanizing racism and *white supremacy*'s brutality are featured throughout.

AMERICAN CHILD PSYCHIATRY: HISTORICAL PERSPECTIVES

For 100 years, we as a people have mourned our great leader [Chief Sitting Bull]. We have followed tradition in our mourning. We have not been happy, have not enjoyed life's beauty, have not danced or sung as a proud nation. . . . Blackness has been around us for one hundred years. During this time the heartbeat of our people has been weak and our lifestyle has deteriorated to a devastating degree.

Box 1
Major conceptual frameworks

Abolition[3]

- Abolition seeks to undo the way of thinking and doing things that see prison and punishment as solutions for all kinds of social, economic, political, behavioral, and interpersonal problems. It calls for defunding the police, removing police from schools, repealing laws that criminalize survival, and providing safe housing for everyone. An act of radical imagination, it demands reorganizing and reimagining and rejects reform.

- Abolition medicine involves constructing new systems of community-based care that challenge the medical-industrial complex rooted in slavery, to build a new, healthier, more just society committed to healing. It reimagines the work of medicine as an antiracist practice; calls for the abolition of race-based diagnostic tools and treatment guidelines that reinforce biological race; and demands longitudinal antiracist training in medical education, desegregating the profession, and reparations for communities devastated by medical experimentation.

Critical race theory (CRT)[55]

- A theoretic framework providing a critical analysis of race and racism to illuminate and combat root causes of structural racism and highlighting the relationship between race, racism, and power.

- Key concepts include: (1) *Ordinariness* (racism and white supremacy in postcivil rights society are integral and normal rather than aberrational); (2) *Centering in the margins* (shifting discourses' starting point from the majority group's perspective—e.g. whiteness—to that of marginalized groups); (3) *Social construction of race* (race was fabricated based on historical, contextual, political considerations); (4) *Intersectionality* (the multidimensionality of oppressions—race, gender identity, class, national origin, sexual orientation—resulting in disempowerment); (5) *Activism:* (commitment to social justice, scholars assume an active role in "eliminating racial oppression as a broad goal of ending all forms of oppression"); (6) *Race consciousness:* (explicit acknowledgment of the workings of race and racism in social contexts or in one's personal life); (7) *Critical consciousness* (digging beneath the surface to develop deeper understandings of concepts, relationships, and personal biases).

Decolonization[56]

- Decolonizing mental health care seeks to heal through culturally-affirming practices and decenters mental health care away from the dominant white, heteronormative, patriarchal, gender-binary narrative.

- It dismantles harmful mental health practices that derive from and reinforce systemic privilege and whiteness. It recognizes the heavily Euro-centric approach to mental health as colonizing and that existing mental health practices do not adequately account for colonization, global issues, and cultural variables. It advances a movement to seek justice and liberation through education, collective care, and activism. It centers the needs of BIPOC and the LGBTQIA2S+ community, honors the full neurodiversity spectrum, and advocates for mental health care accessibility for people with disabilities.

The refusals of white supremacy [15]

- Based on Jamaican philosopher Charles Mills' conception of "the 'epistemology of ignorance' actively maintained by white people to preserve their sense of self as good and the structures preserving their dominance while ignoring the widespread injustice non-white people are forced to suffer to ensure this dominance.

- Five refusals maintain white ignorance: a refusal (1) of the humanity of the other—and a willingness to allow violence and exploitation to be inflicted; (2) to listen to or acknowledge the experience of the other—resulting in marginalization and active silencing; (3) to confront long, violent histories of white domination and to recognize how these continue to shape injustice into the present; (4) to share space, particularly residential space, with resulting segregated geographies that perpetuate inequality and insulate white ignorance.; (5) to face structural causes—capitalism as it has intertwined with white supremacy from its earliest beginnings.

Box 2
Key definitions pertaining to antiracism in child psychiatry

Adultification: a form of dehumanization, robbing Black children of the very essence of what makes childhood distinct from all other developmental periods: innocence. Adultification contributes to a false narrative that Black youths' transgressions are intentional and malicious, instead of the result of immature decision making—a key characteristic of childhood.[17]

Antiracism: Per Ibram X. Kendi, an antiracist idea is any idea that suggests the racial groups are equals in all their apparent differences—that there is nothing right or wrong with any racial group. Antiracist ideas argue that racist policies are the cause of racial inequities. Antiracism is a powerful collection of antiracist policies that lead to racial equity and are substantiated by antiracist ideas.[6]

Carceral logic: refers to the variety of ways our bodies, minds, and actions have been shaped by the idea and practices of imprisonment—even for people who do not see themselves connected explicitly to prisons.[3]

Carceral state: According to Ruby Tapia, (cite needed here) the carceral state encompasses the formal institutions and operations and economies of the criminal justice system proper, but it also encompasses logics, ideologies, practices, and structures, that invest in tangible and sometimes intangible ways in punitive orientations to difference, to poverty, to struggles to social justice and to the crossers of constructed borders of all kinds.[3]

Eugenics: According to psychologist Frances Galton, eugenics is the science which deals with all influences that improve the inborn qualities of a race; also with those that develop them to the utmost advantage. The improvement of the inborn qualities, or stock, of one human population.[19]

Family regulation system: Legal scholar Dorothy Roberts argues that the "child welfare" system, like the "criminal justice" system, is misnamed because it is designed to regulate and punish Black and other marginalized people. It could be more accurately referred to as the "family regulation system."[30]

Historical trauma: cumulative emotional and psychological wounding over the lifespan and across generations, emanating from massive group trauma experiences; the historical trauma response (HTR) is the constellation of features in reaction to this trauma. The HTR often includes depression, self-destructive behavior, suicidal thoughts and gestures, anxiety, low self-esteem, anger, and difficulty recognizing and expressing emotions. It may include substance abuse, often an attempt to avoid painful feelings through self-medication. Historical unresolved grief is the associated effect that accompanies HTR; this grief may be considered fixated, impaired, delayed, and/or disenfranchised.[9]

Intersectionality: the complex, cumulative way for which the effects of multiple forms of discrimination (such as racism, sexism, and classism) combine, overlap, or intersect especially in the experiences of marginalized individuals or groups.[55]

Intergenerational trauma: a phenomenon for which the descendants of a person who has experienced a terrifying event show adverse emotional and behavioral reactions to the event that are similar to those of the person himself or herself.[9]

Medical Industrial Complex: is comprised of interlocking institutions like big pharma, multi-billion dollar health insurance corporations, medical technology companies, and governmental regulatory bodies like the FDA and EPA. These entangled institutions form the basis of US Healthcare and play a profoundly overlooked role in degrading national and global health, perpetuating racism, sexism, classism, homophobia, transphobia, and ableism.[3]

Oppression: "Oppression" refers to a combination of prejudice and institutional power that creates a system that regularly and severely discriminates against some groups and benefits other groups.[57]

Positionality: Positionality refers to how differences in social position and power shape identities and access in society. Citing a few key definitions of positionality, Misawa (2010, p. 26) emphasizes the fluid and relational qualities of social identity formation while also noting that "all parts of our identities are shaped by socially constructed positions and memberships to which we belong" and which are "embedded in our society as a system."

Racial health disparity: Racial and ethnic health and health care disparities refer to the preventable differences in illness and disease, health outcomes, access to and appropriateness of health care seen between minority and nonminority populations.

Reparations: A process of repairing, healing, and restoring people injured because of their group identity and in the violation of their fundamental human rights by governments, corporations, institutions, and families. Those groups that have been injured have the right to obtain from the government, corporation, institution, or family responsible for the injuries that which they need to repair and heal themselves. In addition to being a demand for justice, it is a principle of international human rights law.[4]

Systems of Oppression: The term "systems of oppression" calls attention to the historical and organized patterns of mistreatment. In the US, systems of oppression (like systemic racism) are woven into the very foundation of American culture, society, and laws. Other examples are sexism, heterosexism, ableism, classism, ageism, and anti-Semitism. Society's institutions, such as government, education, and culture, all contribute or reinforce the oppression of marginalized social groups while elevating dominant social groups.[57]

Prison industrial complex (PIC): a term used to describe the overlapping interests of government and industry that use surveillance, policing, and imprisonment as solutions to economic, social, and political problems.[3]

School-to-Prison Pipeline: refers to the school policies and procedures that drive many of our nation's schoolchildren into a pathway that begins in school and ends in the criminal justice system. Black students are suspended and expelled at a rate three times greater than their white peers. Similarly, students with disabilities are more than twice as likely to receive out-of-school suspensions as students with no disabilities and LGBTQ youth are much more likely than their peers to be suspended or expelled.[58]

Settler colonialism: Settler colonialism is a distinct type of colonialism that functions through the replacement of indigenous populations with an invasive settler society that, over time, develops a distinctive identity and sovereignty. Settler colonial states include Canada, the United States, Australia, and South Africa.[59]

Whiteness: A structural apparatus in which that status functions, gains meaning, and adapts over time through laws and norms that empower, normalize, favor, and reward white people as a population. Key aspects of whiteness include:[60]
  White hegemony: establishes and enforces racial hierarchies in which white people nearly exclusively hold decision-making power.[60]
  White normativity: naturalizes power asymmetries between white and non-white people as primarily meritocratic; rests on the idea that white people are the norm while people of color are a deviation from the norm.[60]
  White privilege: preferences white people, actively and passively, by providing and permitting white people disproportionate access to, and benefit from, resources associated with social and economic mobility, such as home-ownership, education, wealth, insurance, and health care.[60]
  White Rage: according to historian Carol Anderson, the enduring historical pattern of white backlash against Black advancement; not infrequently it is violent and deadly.[8]
  White saviorism: when white people "help" minoritized people for selfish reasons—and often end up doing more harm than good—and work from the assumption that they know best what minoritized people need and that it is their responsibility to support and uplift communities of color—in their own country or somewhere else—because minoritized people lack the resources, willpower, and intelligence to do it themselves.[36]
  White supremacy: constructs and maintains a racial ordering of humans and resources that, through various acts of violence or deprivation, justify and enforce the racial dominance of whites.[95]

*Our people now suffer from the highest rates of unemployment, poverty, alco-
holism, and suicide in this country.*
                    —Traditional Hunkpapa Lakota Elders Council (Blackcloud, 1990)

Questions

Why confront child mental health racism by examining its history first? What is the profession's origin story? How has it shaped and been shaped by the legacies of slavery
and *settler colonialism* and their racist, white supremacist, and *carceral logics*? How
does *whiteness* permeate the profession's decades of existence?

Why History Matters

History matters for clinicians embroiled in their professions' legacies and responsible
for reconfiguring their futures and for the lives of patients and families who perpetrate
or bear the weight of centuries of racial violence. Historian Christina Sharpe has
conceptualized slavery's intergenerational effects as living 'in the wake": "to be in
the wake is to occupy and be occupied by the continuous and every changing present
of slavery's as yet unresolved unfolding."[8(pp13-14)] A "past not yet past," slavery
shapes Black people's lived experiences in the present.[8(p13)] Scholar-activist Maria
Yellow Horse Braveheart developed a related concept, *historical trauma*: the cumulative emotional and psychological wounding across generations suffered by indigenous individuals due to *settler colonialism*.[9] Blackcloud's description of the grief
enshrouding his community brings this *intergenerational trauma* to life.
   But what is child psychiatry's relationship to this wake?

American Child Psychiatry in the Wake of Slavery and Settler Colonialism

The wake of slavery courses through child psychiatry's intertwinement with the *carceral
state*. Its early 20th-century beginnings focused on protecting "the normal" by eradi-
cating "maladjusted" behaviors tied to racialized notions of "criminality" and delinquency[10(p329)] Child psychiatry and juvenile courts forged partnerships through child
guidance clinics.[11] "William Healy (1869–1963), who founded the first, The Chicago Juvenile Psychopathic Institute, in 1909, argued that delinquent children had a "psychic
constitutional deficiency."[12] Many came from poor or immigrant families, admitted
based on racist, classist beliefs that they were unable to raise their children "correctly"
for modern, upright society.[11] Although not directly wedded to *eugenics*, these clinics
exalted a white, middle-class ideal. This *white normativity*, in turn, justified incarceration
"as a means of purging. . . and eliminating targeted [minoritized] populations from land,
life, and society in the United States"–including children.[13] Contrasting Black children
enduring a chain gang (**Fig. 1**) with white children reveling atop a pillaged home during
the Red Summer of 1919 (**Fig. 2**) captures how distorted and racist conceptions of "delinquency" were. This white normative orientation sanctioned the racism brutalizing
Black families during Jim Crow and the violence white children perpetrated to sustain it.

AACAP: Steeped in Whiteness

Founded in 1953, AACAP was created primarily by men who ensured their *white hegemony* throughout the 20th century by dominating AACAP presidency and journal
editorship roles. AACAP's original constitution emphasized the subspecialty's medicalized aims and training requirements, while providing zero social justice agenda.
During its first 5 years (1962–1967), the *Journal of the American Academy of Child Psychiatrists* (JAACAP), AACAP's official "voice," made no mention of racism. The 8 out of
10 indigenous children forced into abusive boarding schools settings during this era

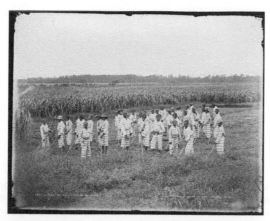

Fig. 1. Spivak, John L. Juvenile convicts at work in the fields. c.1903. Detroit Publishing Company photograph collection, Library of Congress, Washington, D.C. (*From* Spivak, John L. Juvenile convicts at work in the fields. c.1903. Detroit Publishing Company photograph collection, Library of Congress, Washington, D.C.)

carried no valence (**Fig. 3**).[14] The thousands of Black children brutalized by *white rage* when integrating schools were not granted a single breath (**Fig. 4**).[5] The safety and protection of white children was so primary that early issues did not bother distinguishing between white and non-white children, the focus was so inherently dedicated to the former. Against this historical backdrop, AACAP's 2020 response to Jacob Blake's shooting demonstrates, not a commitment to BLM, rather the profession's abiding devotion to the *refusals of white supremacy* (see **Box 1**).[15]

Child Mental Health: Finger-Pointing and White Saviorism

When child psychiatry does begin to concern itself with non-white children, the family emerges as the primary cause behind mental illness and locus of intervention. In the 1970s, juvenile justice shifted from therapeutic, rehabilitative approaches to "deterrence and even retribution."[16(p439)] White child psychiatrists played a key role in this process, pathologizing minoritized families and often recommending children's removal from their homes. As the War on Drugs began ravaging Black families in the 1970s, they indicted poor Black and Brown families, not the racist policies assailing them, unnecessarily exposing children and their families to a racist criminal justice system.[16] This

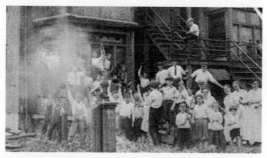

Fig. 2. White children cheer outside an African–American residence that they set on fire, September 1, 1919. Bettman Collection, Getty Images. (*From* White children cheer outside an African-American residence that they set on fire, September 1, 1919. Bettman Collection, Getty Images.)

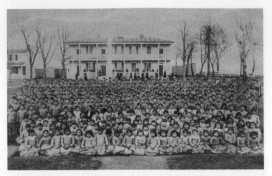

Fig. 3. Pupils at Carlisle Indian Industrial School, Pennsylvania, c. 1900. Carlisle Indian School Digital Resource Center. (*From* Pupils at Carlisle Indian Industrial School, Pennsylvania, c. 1900. Carlisle Indian School Digital Resource Center. Reprinted with permission of Cumberland County Historical Society.)

caused further harm by reinforcing racist ideologies. "Tangle of pathology" stems from the 1965 Moynihan Report about The Negro Family, *adultification* was fabricated during slavery to justify Black children's harsh labor, and both were molded around white children's innocence and normativity. *Adultification* has played a key role in fueling the *school-to-prison pipeline*, while "tangle of pathology" has fueled racist tropes, like "welfare queen," used to undermine public support for the social and family assistance programs.[17–19] Both have devastated generations of non-white children and their communities, reallocating funding and allowing *white privilege* to thrive. As the juvenile justice system gradually moved away from the therapeutic model in the early 1970s, the same judicial flexibility meant to enable rehabilitation and treatment also enabled the disproportionate confinement of children of color."[16(p442)] White child psychiatrists' good intentions when serving minoritized children and families do not exonerate leveraging racialized hierarchies to perpetrate harm—then or now.

Minoritized Families: Overexposure and White Saviorism

Alondra Nelson explains how the Black community in the United States has historically been both *underserved* and *overexposed* to the medical system.[7] The child mental health system—entangled with child protective services, juvenile justice, and public

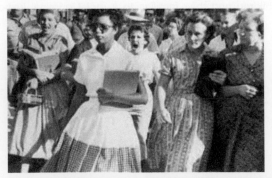

Fig. 4. Elizabeth Eckford ignores the hostile screams and stares of fellow students on her first day of school, September 6, 1957. Bettman Collection, Getty images. (*From* Elizabeth Eckford ignores the hostile screams and stares of fellow students on her first day of school, September 6, 1957. Bettman Collection, Getty images.)

education—overexposes minoritized families to these racist systems, never formally acknowledging potential harm.[20] Early educational programs developed during John-son's 1960s Great Society campaign, like Head Start, depended on "cultural deprivation" theory to justify interventions directed at minoritized children. It conceptualized Black children as deprived of the "normal" stimulating environment white children enjoyed and deficient in their capacity, aptitude, and intellect, relative to white peers. These theories eclipsed any interrogation of interventions' biased practices and metrics of evaluation—including IQ testing, which was highly contested, due to its *eugenic* origins.[21]

Cultural deprivation theory remains part of the wake in child psychiatry. Myriad treatment interventions—similarly developed, researched, and implemented by white clinicians and researchers and practiced on minoritized families—are touted as wholly therapeutic because they fill perceived gaps and deficiencies. Multisystemic therapy (MST) and functional family therapy are 2 examples.[22,23] Their risk of failing to meet or undermining the needs of non-white children is not considered, an oversight more glaring due to their carceral intertwinement.[24] Examples include reducing individual or sibling "recidivism" as a primary treatment outcome and decreasing out of home placements, rather than abolishing the juvenile "injustice" and *family regulation systems* altogether.[25,26] When it comes to child mental health interventions steeped in *whiteness* and *white saviorism* and targeting minoritized families, more (intervention) is always more—even if it causes racist harm.

Throughout the 20th century, the US government kidnapped thousands of indigenous children, forcing them into boarding schools assimilating them to *whiteness* (see **Fig. 3**). These residential schools—centerpieces of "Kill the Indian, Save the man" cultural genocidal policy—paralleled early 20th-century child guidance clinics by upholding *white normativity*. Marking indigenous culture as primitive legitimized killing children, as the hundreds of children's remains recently unearthed in Canada have revealed.[14,27] Other examples of this state-sanctioned family separation rooted in *whiteness* include ripping thousands of children from their parents at the US–Mexico border and generations of Black children from their parents due to slavery and mass incarceration.[28] These histories lay bare the risk of engaging minoritized families in mental healthcare, where Black children are twice as likely as white ones to be reported to child welfare, usually for neglect.[29]

Legal scholar Dorothy Roberts argues that the child welfare system, an integral part of the US carceral regime, should be named the *"family regulation system."* She recommends supplanting it with measures that care for, rather than punish, children and families by addressing upstream causes of neglect, like poverty.[30] Roberts' abolitionist contention contradicts the therapeutic opportunity child maltreatment research interventions presume whenever minoritized families are policed by the family regulation and juvenile injustice systems. SafeCare, an evidence-based parenting curriculum for individuals at risk of or already reported for child maltreatment, is one example. By enhancing parenting and parent–child interactions as core interventions, it turns a blind eye to minoritized families' heightened risk of family separation and trauma related to being policed.[31] The majority of researchers (eg, Greg Aarons, Kate Guastaferro, John Lutzker, Daniel Whitaker) championing it are phenotypically white, manifesting child psychiatry's enduring *white hegemony*.[31–33] SafeCare also represents a contemporary touchpoint for Headstart and other childhood interventions that, beholden to cultural deprivation theory, presume minoritized families' deficiency and salvation through *white saviorism*.[21]

The history of identifying non-white bodies, minds, and feelings as pathologic is also part of this overexposure. Before the 1960s, schizophrenia was a disease often applied to white middle-class women, characterized by docility and emotional disharmony. But during Civil Rights, schizophrenia became defined by aggression and volatility, applied increasingly to Black men engaged in activism.[34] The fenfluramine study conducted in the mid-1990s also focused on biomedical, rather than social, explanations for violence. It administered fenfluramine, now banned for being cardioarrhythmic, to 34 black and Hispanic boys, ages 6 to 10, to prove that their violence and criminality could be predicted by neurotransmitter levels. Endangering minoritized children to prove their predisposition to violence, Mt. Sinai and Columbia vehemently denied any wrongdoing, despite being investigated.[35] American child psychiatry has long recognized the violence of "delinquent" children of color as a public mental health concern—not the structural violence assaulting them—and uplifted white men as chief experts dictating treatment and "care," despite (or perhaps because of) the racist, racialized overtones. The overwhelmingly white researchers leading the fenfluramine study is one example.[35] The entirely white and predominantly male working committee behind AACAP's 1997 "Practice Parameter for the Assessment and Treatment of Children with Conduct Disorder," yet another.[36] One committee member, Dr William Ayres, was later convicted of molesting his child patients after serving as AACAP president, raising grave concerns about the profession's white (patriarchal) hegemony's own risk of aggression.[37]

These examples recall diagnoses like "drapetomania" that categorized runaway slaves as ill, rather than the white people perpetrating daily violence against them. They conjure the dangerous treatments 19th-century white male physicians prescribed, such as whipping to "treat" drapetomania, maintaining the *systems of oppression* they dominated, continuing the rape and plunder, watching the cash come in.[34] Pathologizing minoritized people's feelings as biomedical, innate difference, rather than an adaptive response to this cruelty, reveals how psychiatric diagnoses have been weaponized against Black and Brown populations. The overdiagnosis of oppositional defiant disorder and conduct disorder among minoritized children represents one contemporary touchpoint.[38] The firewater myth, the pervasive false belief that indigenous individuals use alcohol at higher rates are biologically more vulnerable to alcohol problems, represents another. A tool of colonization, it falsely incriminates indigenous individuals for "disproportionately" consuming alcohol, distracting from their heightened vulnerabilities to the consequences of alcohol use, due to the structural legacy of *settler colonialism*—disproportionately constructed by white colonizers.[39]

Minoritized Families: Underserved and Deserving of Social Health

Nelson's history of sickle cell anemia illustrates how a disease disproportionately impacting people of African descent was disregarded and underfunded *because* of whom it impacted most.[7] Herein lies the paradox of the medical system's (mis)treatment of Black bodies and minds: if they are not considered diseased and therefore overexposed to medicine, their health concerns are diminished or ignored, and they are underserved by medicine. This neglect reflects the "wake" of slavery, undervaluing Black suffering and maintaining theories of "racial resistance" and racial difference.[40] Claiming Black bodies were "stronger" and more impervious to hard labor and painful punishments validated white slaveholders violent practices.[19] Claiming that white bodies and minds were more violent and sociopathic—demonstrated by their capacity to monetize and dehumanize Black bodies—were never made. Child psychiatry's focus on resilience among minoritized youth echoes this racial resistance concept, suggesting their unique ability to live with and thrive in the face of oppression is a sign of wellbeing, rather than violence they have no choice but to suffer. Resilience discourses conveniently shift the locus of responsibility for dismantling *systems of oppression* away from the profession, exonerating it for upholding it. Not surprisingly, many of JAACAP's most recent articles pertaining to resilience in non-white children were lead-authored by white men.[41–43] The *white hegemony* of organized child psychiatry's early years reverberates, rigging discourses, maintaining racial hierarchies, and thwarting the *antiracist* action needed for transformative change.

History implores us to move toward what Nelson terms "social health": scaling individual well-being to the well-being of the body politic and attending to *social* explanations for health inequities, rather than scientific or biomedical ones. In the 1960s, Frantz Fanon, a psychiatrist from Martinique, argued that neuroses and psychopathologies in colonized populations were products of the political and social forces of the colonizer. This logic challenged justifying narratives for imperial control, namely that the colonized population was pathologic, diseased and naturally incapable of governing themselves. It offered an alternative social explanation for neuroses in the Black colonized subject, perpetrated by the white colonizer.[44] American scientific racism borrowed heavily from these colonial logics. The idea of non-white subjects having "primitive" minds needing the care and direction of white (male) experts aligns with the histories detailed here. We must move toward a more holistic, socially informed psychiatry that acknowledges the devastating health consequences from the legacies of *white supremacy*.

But before reimagining the future, the present must be reckoned with.

PAINTING THE LANDSCAPE OF CONTEMPORARY RACIST INEQUITIES

It would be easy to speculate about the impact of years of cocaine use on my father's heart, but I suspect that it will tell us less than if we could measure the cumulative effects of hatred, racism, and indignity. What is the impact of years of strip searches, or being bent over, the years before that when you were a child and knew that no dream you had for yourself was taken seriously by anyone, that you were not someone who would be fully invested in by a nation that treated you as expendable. What is the impact of not being valued? How do you measure the loss of what a human being does not receive?
   —*BLM Founder Patrisse Khan-Cullors reflecting on her father, who "died of a broken heart in a nation of broken promises"*[45]

Questions

How do racism and *white supremacy* intersect with other *systems of oppression* to impact child mental health today? Do our existing measures capture the enormity of this toll? Can epidemiologic findings help us reimagine the practice of child mental health as an *antiracist* one? How do we tell the story of racism's impact on child mental health more fully to fulfill the mandate for an *antiracist* present and future?

The Problem with Racial Disparities: a Refusal of White Supremacy

In the realm of (child) mental health, "*racial disparities*," a dominant framework describing racism, provides an instructive example of how related frameworks—like cultural humility and the social determinants of health—fail to enliven racism's magnitude. Diagnoses and access to mental health treatment represent the primary outcomes. Studies indicate that while minoritized children have a similar or lower prevalence of mental disorders compared with white children, they are more likely than white people to have severe and persistent mental disorders and less likely to access mental health care.[46–48] Highlighting these population-level differences presumes these diagnoses are accurate, objective markers of emotional health for all children and that child mental health care is universally safe and therapeutic.

But centering racism's well-established devastating impact on child mental health and invoking its history of racism yield diametrically opposed interpretations: these diagnoses are racialized, racist measures of suffering for minoritized individuals actively refusing to enter a mental health system whereby they face a great risk of discrimination and harm. This risk is manifested in misdiagnosis, coercive "care," assessment tools normed to *whiteness*, loss of civil liberties, and being overreported to child protective services.[29,38,49] It is personified in the murder of Daniel Prude, who was discharged from a reputable psychiatric emergency room, only to be lynched by the police while psychotic later the same day.[50] Invoking a *CRT framework* helps interrogate the *positionality* of leading experts shaping the racial disparities framework, inviting important questions about their intersecting axes of power and privilege. It questions their ability to shape this discourse in an *antiracist* fashion while sequestered in ivory towers, alienated from the masses whose needs they claim to center.

The language of "disparities" condones skimming the surface of centuries-long *white supremacist* violence while erasing the *intergenerational trauma* minoritized communities have suffered as a result. Static in nature and ahistorical by design, it implies that racial "differences" are something to be observed; the historical violence giving rise to them, buried in denial. "Disproportionality" may be applied to Black children's increased likelihood of living in poorer, segregated neighborhoods and Black mothers' increased risk of dying during childbirth.[51] But refusing to link these statistics to the failures of 40 acres and a mule and the sexual violence foundational to American slavery represents active denial of the atrocities giving rise to these numbers, absolving the profession's responsibility to engage in historically oriented repair. Its willful ignorance constitutes a violation of the oath to first do no harm, one that child psychiatry, nearly exclusive in its service to white children, has never acknowledged. Disparities' descriptive, ahistorical nature cultivates a spectator role for the profession, forcing a sharp turn away from immediate antiracist action. Standards of care cannot mandate challenging racist violence when a prevailing discourse solely requires providers to stare at and describe it. Emphasizing differences along the socially fabricated fault lines of race risks reinforcing biological racial differences while naturalizing them as constant and unchangeable. Similar shortcomings pertain to cultural humility and the social determinants of health. If a framework does not report the state violence and *white supremacy* causing harm, it cannot possibly mandate antiracist repair.

Conceptual models pertaining to child mental health disparities emphasize socioeconomic status (eg, low education and income), childhood adversities (eg, maltreatment, family violence), and family structure across development (eg, single motherhood, early child-bearing).[52] The professional corpus reifies the wake by first turning its back away from the centuries of white supremacist violence and next, pointing the finger of blame toward minoritized families brutalized by it. Interventions addressing racial health disparities make no mention of antioppressive measures, like dismantling structural *whiteness* or seeking reparations. They do not imagine nor mandate antiracist approaches curbing the pro-white implicit bias harming children's developmental trajectories during clinical care.[20] This narrative script forged through lies the profession tells itself ultimately fortifies racial hierarchies of all types. The professional elites rigging the discourses pertaining to racism in (child) mental health see their power unchanged by a framework that describes, not dismantles, the *systems of oppression* benefiting them. Minoritized individuals seeking care endure blame and pathologizing for their suffering at the hands of unchallenged *white supremacy*. The past of American child psychiatry, steeped in *whiteness*, endures in the present.

Reconfiguring Racial Disparities as Racist Inequities Rooted in History

Racial disparities pertaining to diagnostic criteria and access to mental health care cannot capture racism and *white supremacy*'s devastating impact on child mental health. Doing so requires a comprehensive approach that incorporates intergenerational, historical, and intersectional perspectives accounting for other *systems of oppression*, like cissexism and heterosexism; multi-level understandings of racism; and multi-disciplinary approaches incorporating history and other social sciences. Spanning centuries and probing root causes, this expansive analysis honors racism's complexity and rejects sanitized frameworks maintaining the status quo. Rooted in *CRT*, *abolition*, and *decolonization* (see **Box 1**), it lubricates the gearshift for meaningful *antiracism* mandates of the profession. Performative diversity and inclusion initiatives committed to stalling transformational change crumble like a house of cards. A new unimagined approach transcends the "violence of abstraction" exacted by statistical analyses.[8] The personal—stories, memoir, and narrative—serve as a portal into the social and historical processes that birthed these numbers in the first place. It's time to begin to imagine an antiracist present and future in child psychiatry by first confronting and naming its deep-seeded racist inequities.

What would this vision of the future look like in our ancestors' wildest dreams?

DISCUSSION AND SUMMARY: IMAGINING AN ANTIRACIST PRESENT AND FUTURE

Historically, pandemics have forced humans to break with the past and imagine their world anew. This one is no different. It is a portal, a gateway between one world and the next. We can choose to walk through it, dragging the carcasses of our prejudice and hatred, our avarice, our data banks and dead ideas, our dead rivers and smoky skies behind us. Or we can walk through lightly, with little luggage, ready to imagine another world. And ready to fight for it.

—Arundhati Roy, 2020[53]

Questions

What would it take to disrupt the legacy of racism and white supremacy in American child psychiatry? How would we get there? How would we know when we arrived? What are the better questions we can ask to galvanize a movement that overcomes the existing sanitized frameworks cementing our inertia? How do we serve the children—all the children—body and soul? Who is at the table making decisions for the profession? What does accountability look like for those in power?

Serving Children's Mental Health Body and Soul: Confronting a Racist Past to Reimagine an Antiracist Future

April 2021. Say her name: Ma'Khia Bryant (2005–2021). Her life embodies how racism—in Ruth Wilson Gilmore's words—represents "the 'state-sanctioned or extralegal production and exploitation of group-differentiated vulnerability to premature death.'[3] Shot by a white Columbus, Ohio police officer, the carceral state stole her life at age 16 minutes before Derek Chauvin's verdict was announced.[54] She embodied the 50% of Black children reported to child protective services, in her case for neglect, and the disproportionate number of Black children in foster care.[29] She cycled through 5 placements, while her grandmother struggled to regain custody, which she lost due to insecure housing—herself the victim of the enduring legacy of redlining and segregation.[54] On the day her sister called 911 begging for adults to "protect and serve," Ma'Khia was adultified, dehumanized, labeled the aggressor, and shot four times. Mayor Andrew Ginther commented, "Some of us are guilty, but all of us are responsible." Similar to Trayvon Martin and Tamir Rice, AACAP said nothing. Nothing about policing, race-based traumatic stress, the *family regulation system*, or *adultification*. This is the evidence base for how racist inequities seeded centuries ago continue to wreak havoc.

2022. Galvanized by Ma'Khia Bryant's murder, child psychiatry commits to reversing the wake of slavery and settler colonialism. The guiding question: how could this profession have assumed responsibility for preventing this child's death; and in its failure, what does accountability to Ma'Khia, her family, and community look like? The answer: a movement that takes form in a special committee assembled by the next generation of child psychiatrists with expertise—lived and otherwise—in racism and antiracism. It includes child mental health providers promoting the *decolonization* of mental health, historians of medicine, children and families who have survived the *medical industrial complex*, and community organizations and legal scholars committed to *abolition*. Through monthly town halls, the collective determines the most pressing antiracist needs for children and families overlooked since AACAP's founding in 1953. Embracing Roy's metaphor of the pandemic as a portal, they "break with the past and imagine[s] their world anew," establishing key priorities for clinical care, public health activism, research, and the antiracist training of child psychiatry fellows. The original AACAP constitution is rewritten and entitled "A New Constitution for an Antiracist Future."

2027. The child mental health antiracist collective has flourished. The history of child mental health and antiracist clinical care sub-committees has developed a truth and reconciliation process for uncovering child psychiatry's perpetuation of the wake of slavery and *settler colonialism*. They report their findings to the public as a form of accountability and atonement and emphasize the profession's *refusals of white supremacy*, its white hegemonic rigging of discourses, and its overexposure and undertreatment of minoritized children and families. They identify contemporary clinical practices linked to this uninterrogated history and dialogue about whether to abolish or reform them.

The child psychiatrists who formed the collective in 2022 mentor the next wave of child psychiatrists, cultivating their fresh insights and perspectives. In 5 years, they developed *antiracism* guidelines for research, clinical care, and training and submitted recommendations to ACGME to establish *antiracism* as a competency—one that rejects cultural humility because it cultivates the practices that would have prevented Ma Khia's death. They created an antiracist algorithm to interrogate the racism and *white supremacy* permeating AACAP guidelines, position statements, and other "evidence-based" treatment interventions. It commodifies and explicitly states their risk of racist harm and names their creators' positionality as part of their informed and consented use. They innovate a new framework naming racist inequities rooted in history to dismantle them. Frameworks like *CRT*, *abolition*, and *decolonization* guide their efforts. No longer drowning in *whiteness*, child psychiatry begins to transcend it.

Their organizing and activism are not universally well-received. The *white hegemony* of the profession, undeterred since 1953, claims that the new approaches are not "evidence-based" or "scientific" and demands data to back the movement's efforts and quantify its impact. They argue that dismantling evidence-based mental health interventions with carceral links is "anti-psychiatry." The antiracist collective, having unpacked the profession's long-standing *refusals of white supremacy*, anticipated this resistance in 2022 and strategically side-steps it. Refusing to engage in "faculty development" and continuing medical education processes for those deeply tied to a racist, white supremacist past, it divests from the establishment, reinvesting in the antiracist collective' accountability to the public. The movement continues to grow.

2032. Ten years later, efforts to abolish the family regulation and juvenile injustice systems are gaining traction. Child psychiatry has become part of the vanguard of medical specialties defining and innovating *abolition medicine*.[4] It is actively being reimagined as an antiracist practice for the people. The number of minoritized physicians pursuing child psychiatry fellowship soars to record numbers. Finally seeing a place for themselves and for their families in this profession, they believe in playing a key role to shape it. The antiracist collective has implemented policy changes banning all-white teams from researching minoritized children and families or creating interventions and practice parameters to treat them. The risk of harm is too great. Massive shifts in child global mental health and child welfare research emerge as a result.

Ma'Khia Bryant's spirit lives on in the ongoing creation of a healing profession that nurtures all of childrens', bodies and souls. The possibilities for the future are limitless.

CLINICS CARE POINTS

- Antiracist child mental health care challenges the profession's longstanding refusals of white supremacy by ensuring diagnostic and treatment practices challenge, rather than uphold, violent histories of white domination.
- Antiracist child mental health care requires examining the danger of overexposing minoritized children and families to child mental health care and increasing their risk of being policed by the family regulation and other carceral systems.
- Antiracist child mental health care considers the risk of perpetuating cultural deprivation's "wake" by presuming deficiencies among minoritized children and families that can only be filled by interventions created by white people.
- Antiracism child mental health care identifies the risk of normalizing white rage and racial violence and prioritizing white innocence over minoritized suffering.
- Clinicians can apply abolition, Critical Race Theory, and decolonization frameworks to their care by avoiding punitive, coercive, carceral practices; recognizing racism and white supremacy's pervasiveness; and decentering white cisheteronormativity as a marker of health and wellbeing.

DISCLOSURE

The authors have no conflicts of interest to disclose. They collectively contributed hundreds of hours and centuries of lived experience. In the process, they endured retraumatization while confronting white supremacist violence and risking censure from their employers and institutions for their unapologetic, transparent approach. The emotional, intellectual, and physical toll of this labor on their bodies cannot be quantified. The only remuneration they received for their free labor was support from one another. While invaluable, this is also unacceptable. The motivation for their unpaid contribution is that it serves as an impetus and mandate to fund long overdue and desperately needed anti-racism initiatives in American child psychiatry.

REFERENCES

1. AACAP. AACAP responds to police shooting of Mr. Jacob Blake, Kenosha, Wisconsin. Available at: https://www.aacap.org/AACAP/Latest_News/AACAP_response_police_shooting_jacob_blake.aspx. Accessed September 11, 2021.
2. Buchanan L, Bui Q, Patel JK. Black lives matter may be the largest movement in U.S. history. The New York Times; 2020. Available at: https://www.nytimes.com/interactive/2020/07/03/us/george-floyd-protests-crowd-size.html. Accessed September 11, 2021.
3. Kaba M, Murakawa N. We do this' til we free us: abolitionist organizing and transforming justice. Chicago: Haymarket Books; 2021.
4. Iwai Y, Khan ZH, DasGupta S. Abolition medicine. Lancet 2020;396:158–9.
5. Anderson C. White rage: the unspoken truth of our racial divide. New York: Bloomsbury Publishing USA; 2016.
6. Kendi IX. How to be an antiracist. New York: Random House Publishing Group; 2019.

7. Nelson A. Body and soul: the Black Panther Party and the fight against medical discrimination. Minneapolis: U of Minnesota Press; 2011.

8. Sharpe C. In the wake: on blackness and being. Durham: Duke University Press; 2016.

9. Heart B, Horse MY. Wakiksuyapi: carrying the historical trauma of the Lakota. Tul Stud Soc Welfare 2000;21:245–66.

10. Filipe AM. The rise of child psychiatry in Portugal: an intimate social and political history, 1915–1959. Soc Hist Med 2014;27:326–48.

11. Jones KW. Taming the troublesome child: American families, child guidance, and the limits of psychiatric authority. Cambridge: Harvard University Press; 1999.

12. Earls F. Oppositional-defiant and conduct disorders. In: Rutter MT, Hersov EA, editors. Child and adolescent psychiatry: modern approaches. Oxford: Blackwell Scientific; 1994. p. 308–29.

13. Hernández KL. City of inmates: conquest, rebellion, and the rise of human caging in Los Angeles, 1771–1965. Chapel Hill: UNC Press Books; 2017.

14. NABS. Kill the Indian, save the man:" an introduction to the history of boarding schools. 2020. Available at: https://boardingschoolhealing.org/kill-the-indian-save-the-man-an-introduction-to-the-history-of-boarding-schools/. Accessed October 2, 2021.

15. Gibbons A. The five refusals of white supremacy. Am J Econ Sociol 2018;77:729–55.

16. Raz M. Psychiatrists and the transformation of juvenile justice in Philadelphia, 1965–1972. J Hist Med Allied Sci 2018;73:437–63.

17. Epstein R, Blake J, González T. Girlhood interrupted: the erasure of Black girls' childhood. 2017. Available at: https://papers.ssrn.com/sol3/papers.cfm?abstract_id=3000695. Accessed October 3, 2021.

18. Moynihan DP. The Negro family: the case for national action. Washington, DC: Office of Planning and Research; 1965.

19. Kendi IX. From the beginning: the definitive history of racist ideas in America. New York City: Nation Books; 2016.

20. Harris M, Benton H. Implicit bias in the child welfare, education and mental health systems. National Center for Youth Law. Available at: http://www.centerforchildwelfare.org/kb/cultcomp/Implicit-Bias-in-Child-Welfare-Education-and-Mental-Health-Systems-Literature-Review_061915.pdf. Accessed October 3, 2021.

21. Raz M. What's wrong with the poor?: psychiatry, race, and the War on Poverty. Chapel Hill: UNC Press Books; 2013.

22. Schoenwald SK, Heiblum N, Saldana L, et al. The international implementation of multisystemic therapy. Eval Health Prof 2008;31:211–25.

23. Alexander JF. Functional family therapy. American Psychological Association. Available at: https://www.apa.org/pubs/videos/4310782. Accessed October 3, 2021.

24. Bunting A, Fox S, Adhyaru J, et al. Considerations for minority ethnic young people in multisystemic therapy. Clin Child Psychol Psychiatry 2021;26:268–82.

25. Wagner DV, Borduin CM, Sawyer AM, et al. Long-term prevention of criminality in siblings of serious and violent juvenile offenders: a 25-year follow-up to a randomized clinical trial of multisystemic therapy. J Consult Clin Psychol 2014;82:492–9.

26. Johnides BD, Borduin CM, Wagner DV, et al. Effects of multisystemic therapy on caregivers of serious juvenile offenders: a 20-year follow-up to a randomized clinical trial. J Consult Clin Psychol 2017;85:323–34.

27. Austen I. "Horrible history": mass grave of Indigenous children reported in Canada. The New York Times; 2021. Available at: https://www.nytimes.com/2021/05/28/world/canada/kamloops-mass-grave-residential-schools.html. Accessed October 3, 2021.

28. Miranda J, Legha R. The consequences of family separation at the border and beyond. J Am Acad Child Adolesc Psychiatry 2019;58:139–40.

29. Kim H, Wildeman C, Jonson-Reid M, et al. Lifetime prevalence of investigating child maltreatment among US children. Am J Public Health 2017;107:274–80.

30. Roberts D. Abolishing policing also means abolishing family regulation. The Imprint. 2020. Available at: https://imprintnews.org/child-welfare-2/abolishing-policing-also-means-abolishing-family-regulation/44480#:~:text=It%20could%20be%20more%20accurately,and%20control%20of%20black%20communities. Accessed October 3, 2021.

31. Guastaferro KM, Lutzker JR, Graham ML, et al. SafeCare®: historical perspective and dynamic development of an evidence-based scaled-up model for the prevention of child maltreatment. Psychosoc Interv 2012;21:171–80.

32. Fettes DL, Sklar M, Green AE, et al. Racial and ethnic differences in depressive profiles of child welfare–involved families receiving home visitation services. Psychiatr Serv 2021;72:539–45.

33. Whitaker DJ, Ryan KA, Wild RC, et al. Initial implementation indicators from a statewide rollout of SafeCare within a child welfare system. Child Maltreat 2012;17:96–101.

34. Metzl JM. The protest psychosis: how schizophrenia became a Black disease. Boston: Beacon Press; 2010.

35. Shamoo AE, Tauer CA. Ethically questionable research with children: the fenfluramine study. Account Res 2002;9:143–66.

36. Steiner H. Practice parameters for the assessment and treatment of children and adolescents with conduct disorder. J Am Acad Child Adolesc Psychiatry 1997; 36:122S.

37. Examiner Staff. Ex-psychiatrist William Ayres gets 8 years in prison for child molestations. The san Francisco examiner. 2013. Available at: https://www.sfexaminer.com/news/ex-psychiatrist-william-ayres-gets-8-years-in-prison-for-child-molestations/. Accessed October 3, 2021.

38. Fadus MC, Odunsi OT, Squeglia LM. Race, ethnicity, and culture in the medical record: implicit bias or patient advocacy? Acad Psychiatry 2019;43:532–6.

39. Beauvais F. American Indians and alcohol. Alcohol Health Res World 1998;22:253–9.

40. Crenner C. The Tuskegee Syphilis Study and the scientific concept of racial nervous resistance. J Hist Med Allied Sci 2012;67:244–80.

41. Austin JL, Jeffries EF, Winston W, et al. Race-related stressors and resources for resilience: associations with emotional health, conduct problems, and academic investment among African American early adolescents. J Am Acad Child Adolesc Psychiatry 2021. https://doi.org/10.1016/j.jaac.2021.05.020.

42. Moshofsky SA. 49.1 Building resilience in young women rescued from sexual trafficking in Indonesia. J Am Acad Child Adolesc Psychiatry 2020;59:S245.

43. Biel MG, Hamrah O. Learning from the pandemic:" building back better" through research on risk and resilience with diverse populations. J Am Acad Child Adolesc Psychiatry 2021;. https://pesquisa.bvsalud.org/controlecancer/resource/pt/mdl-33581228?src=similardocs.

44. Fanon F. The wretched of the earth. New York City: Grove/Atlantic, Inc; 2007.

45. Cullors P, Bandele A. When they call you a terrorist: a Black Lives Matter memoir. New York City: St. Martin's Publishing Group; 2018.

46. Cook BL, Hou SS-Y, Lee-Tauler SY, et al. A review of mental health and mental health care disparities research: 2011-2014. Med Care Res Rev 2019;76:683–710.

47. Lu W. Treatment for adolescent depression: national patterns, temporal trends, and factors related to service use across settings. J Adolesc Health 2020;67: 401–8.

48. Lu W. Child and adolescent mental disorders and health care disparities: results from the National Survey of Children's Health, 2011–2012. J Health Care Poor Underserved 2017;28:988–1011.

49. Nash KA, Tolliver DG, Taylor RA, et al. Racial and Ethnic disparities in physical restraint use for pediatric patients in the emergency department. JAMA Pediatr 2021. https://doi.org/10.1001/jamapediatrics.2021.3348.

50. Dahlberg B. Rochester hospital released Daniel Prude hours before fatal encounter with police. NPR; 2020. Available at: https://www.npr.org/sections/health-shots/2020/09/29/917317141/rochester-hospital-released-daniel-prude-hours-before-fatal-encounter-with-polic. Accessed October 2, 2021.

51. TCF. Attacking the Black–white opportunity gap that comes from residential segregation. 2019. Available at;. https://tcf.org/content/report/attacking-black-white-opportunity-gap-comes-residential-segregation/?agreed=1Published June 25. Accessed October 2, 2021.

52. Alegría M, Green JG, McLaughlin KA, et al. Disparities in child and adolescent mental health and mental health services in the US. New York City: William T Grant Foundation; 2015.

53. Roy A. The pandemic is a portal. Financ Times; 2020. Available at: https://www.paxchristi.org.au/wp-content/uploads/2020/07/Disarming-Times-Vol-45-No-2-1.pdf. Accessed October 3, 2021.

54. Bogel-Burroughs N, Barry E, Wright W. Ma'Khia Bryant's journey through foster care ended with an officer's bullet. The New York Times; 2021. Available at: https://www.nytimes.com/2021/05/08/us/columbus-makhia-bryant-foster-care.html. Accessed October 3, 2021.

55. Ford CL, Airhihenbuwa CO. Critical race theory, race equity, and public health: toward antiracism praxis. Am J Public Health 2010;100(Suppl 1):S30–5.

56. Fellner KD. Returning to our medicines: decolonizing and Indigenizing mental health services to better serve Indigenous communities in urban spaces. 2016. Available at: https://open.library.ubc.ca/collections/83l/24/items/1.0228859. Accessed October 3, 2021.

57. NMAAHC. Social identities and systems of oppression. 2019. Available at: https://nmaahc.si.edu/learn/talking-about-race/topics/social-identities-and-systems-oppression. Accessed October 3, 2021.

58. ADL. What is the school-to-prison oipeline? Available at: https://www.adl.org/education/educator-resources/lesson-plans/what-is-the-school-to-prison-pipeline. Accessed October 4, 2021.

59. Bhambra G. Settler colonialism. Available at: https://globalsocialtheory.org/concepts/settler-colonialism/. Published August 4, 2015. Accessed October 4, 2021.

60. Boyd RW. The case for desegregation. Lancet 2019;393:2484–5.

Striving for Equity in Community Mental Health: Opportunities and Challenges for Integrating Care for BIPOC Youth

Eric Rafla-Yuan, MD[a],*, Shavon Moore, MD[b],
Hernán Carvente-Martinez, BSc[c], Phillip Yang, MA[d],
Lilanthi Balasuriya, MD[e], Kamilah Jackson, MD, MPH[f],
Courtney McMickens, MD, MPH, MHS[g],
Barbara Robles-Ramamurthy, MD[h]

KEYWORDS

- Collaborative care • Integrated care • Child mental health • BIPOC
- Community mental health • Racism • Childhood trauma • Advocacy

KEY POINTS

- For BIPOC youth, the vulnerability of minors intersects with racism, worsening mental health, access to health care, and nearly every other outcome
- Integrating psychiatric care into general medical settings has emerged as an evidence based method to address the lack of access to psychiatric care for children and adolescents
- To effectively reach BIPOC youth, care must extend beyond medical settings to other child-focused sectors, including local governments, education, child welfare, and juvenile legal systems
- Intentional policy decisions are needed to incentivize and support these systems, which typically rely on coordination and collaboration between clinicians and other stakeholders
- Clinicians must be trauma-informed and structurally competent to successfully navigate and advocate for collaborative systems that benefit BIPOC youth

[a] Department of Psychiatry, University of California San Diego, 9500 Gilman Drive, #0851, San Diego, CA 92093, USA; [b] Department of Psychiatry, UC San Diego Health Psychiatry – La Jolla, 8950 Villa La Jolla Drive, Suite C101, MC 9057, La Jolla, CA 92037, USA; [c] Healing Ninjas, Inc., 85-04 113th Street, Apt 2, Richmond Hill, NY 11418, USA; [d] Joe R. and Teresa Lozano Long School of Medicine, University of Texas Health San Antonio, 7703 Floyd Curl Drive, MC 7985, San Antonio, TX 78229, USA; [e] Yale University School of Medicine, 333 Cedar Street, SHM IE-66, PO Box 208088, New Haven, CT 06510-8088, USA; [f] PerformCare, 300 Horizon Drive Suit 306, Trenton, NJ 08691, USA; [g] North Carolina, Eleanor Health, 610 Pembroke Road, Greensboro, NC 27408-7608, USA; [h] Department of Psychiatry and Behavioral Sciences, University of Texas Health San Antonio, 7703 Floyd Curl Drive, MC 7792, San Antonio, TX 78229, USA
* Corresponding author.
E-mail address: eraflayuan@ucsd.edu

Child Adolesc Psychiatric Clin N Am 31 (2022) 295–312
https://doi.org/10.1016/j.chc.2021.11.007
1056-4993/22/© 2021 Elsevier Inc. All rights reserved.

INTRODUCTION

If we are going to be intentional about developing policies aimed at improving care that youth and families receive, then we must also continuously partner with them to ensure that systems and policies are being created with their experiences in mind. I don't want to keep seeing other youth fall through the cracks like I did.
—Hernán Carvente-Martinez

Supporting the mental health of youth who identify as Black, Indigenous, or Persons of Color (BIPOC) continues to be a challenge for clinicians and policymakers alike.[1] Children and adolescents are a vulnerable population, with development influenced by numerous environmental and familial factors. For BIPOC youth, these vulnerabilities are magnified by the effects of racism in all its forms, including policies leading to higher rates of housing instability, nutritional insecurity, incarceration, and illness, among many others.[2] Alarmingly, recent data show a disproportionate increase in rates of psychiatric illness among BIPOC youth, including deaths from suicide.[3] These increases are particularly startling among Black youth, bringing an urgency for clinicians and policymakers alike to address this public health threat.[4,5]

Integration of psychiatric care into other medical or community settings has emerged as an evidence-based method to address the lack of access to psychiatric

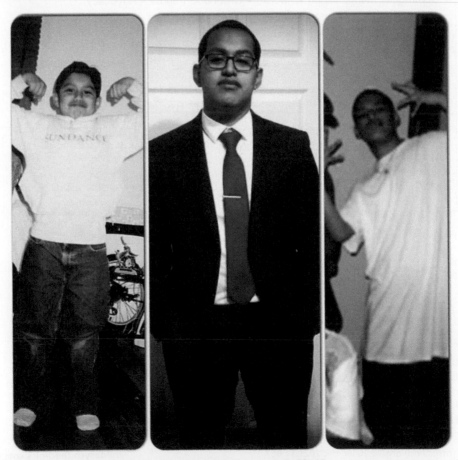

Fig. 1. The Journey of Hernán Carvente-Martinez: ages 9, 23, 15.

care for children and adolescents.[6] However, to bridge the gap experienced by BIPOC youth, care must extend beyond general pediatric medical settings to other child-focused sectors, including local governments, education, child welfare, and juvenile legal systems. Intentional policy decisions are needed to support these developments. In this article, we review some of the opportunities and challenges for integrating mental health care for BIPOC youth (**Fig. 1**).

Living Clinical Case Study

Hernán is a 29-year-old social entrepreneur and advocate for prison abolition (**Fig. 1**). His life story demonstrates a pattern of circumstances experienced by many youth who end up in the juvenile legal system. We purposefully choose to not call it the juvenile justice system because the evidence available does not demonstrate that justice is served by this system. Hernán was born in the United States (US) but his family moved to Mexico when he was 3 year old. He lived in Mexico from ages 3–8, experiencing physical violence from his father, witnessing heavy alcohol consumption by his father and domestic violence between his parents, and experiencing sexual abuse by a neighbor. Growing up, he never spoke to anyone about these experiences, and moved back to the US at age 8, unknowingly as a U.S. citizen within a mixed-status family. Hernán also began consuming alcohol at age 8, believing as a child that if he drank the remaining alcohol first, there would not be enough for his father to get drunk. As a teenager, Hernán was described as displaying "aggressive behaviors" and was defensive when adults attempted to connect with him. He joined a gang and began using cocaine by age 14. At 15, Hernán and his girlfriend had a child on the way. In his neighborhood, Hernán felt authorities at school saw him as a criminal, which was reinforced when police officers repeatedly used excessive force when interacting with him. Through gang-related activities and at the age of 16, Hernán was charged with attempted murder. It was not until 2017 that New York State raised the age of criminal responsibility to 18, so he was fortunate to be remanded to a juvenile, rather than adult, correctional facility. He finally began receiving basic mental health services while in juvenile correctional facilities, but he was typically offered medication rather than therapy, support, or connection. The repeating trauma Hernán experienced and witnessed worsened his mental status and continued to limit his ability to connect with others.

It was not until after a high-risk suicide attempt in his late twenties that Hernán again accessed mental health services. By connecting with other members of his own community, and pursuing social connections in addition to therapy and traditional psychiatric treatment, he has begun his recovery process. Throughout this article, you will find quotes from Hernán describing opportunities and challenges for expanding and integrating care for BIPOC youth and families.

BACKGROUND & DEFINITIONS
BIPOC Youth and the Sociopolitical Determinants of Health

I am Mexican, Brown, and the son of undocumented immigrants. I deserve mental health care just as much as a white person in my community.

BIPOC, referring to *Black, Indigenous, and other Persons of Color*, first emerged in 2013 as an attempt to center historically marginalized Black and Indigenous individuals in larger discussions on racism and equity.[7] By definition, the term BIPOC attempts to encapsulate all non-white persons, an extremely heterogeneous and dissimilar grouping. We acknowledge limitations in terminology and data as studied thus far, and attempt to review the existing knowledge base in a manner informed by historic and ongoing work detailing how currently existing systems have been designed and governed based on white supremacist principles.[8,9]

White supremacy and structurally racist policy decisions have had lasting effects on the health of numerous generations of BIPOC youth.[10,11] Racism is defined by the

CDC as, "a system of structuring opportunity and assigning value based on race,"[12] and can be defined in structural, interpersonal, and internalized terms.[13] Structural racism, often manifesting through the sociopolitical determinants of health, decreases both quality and access to care, while simultaneously increasing risk factors for psychiatric illness. Interpersonal racism, including bias and discrimination between individuals, occurs consciously and unconsciously. Internalized racism refers to conscious and unconscious acceptance of white supremacist principles.[2,12,14] All levels of racism detrimentally impact BIPOC youth, worsening mental health outcomes.[9,14–16]

"When we think of the present mental health narrative, it wasn't one that I could relate to because it doesn't actively include the demographic, cultural, orcommunity-centeredlanguage that connects with me as a young Latinx mental health organizer who has been impacted by incarceration, childhood trauma, community violence, and so many other challenges. I grew up seeing mental health as something that was only forwhite-identifyingpeople. I experienced my parents, community, and immediate support system turning to the police before they considered turning to a therapist or counselor—it just wasn't accessible to people who looked like me."

It is important for clinicians to understand that BIPOC youth do not have a biological predisposition to mental illness, which has been previously used as a false medical narrative to explain disproportionate negative outcomes in BIPOC populations. Rather, these differences stem from societal and environmental factors, which are neither coincidental nor naturally occurring phenomena.[10] For BIPOC youth and families, outcomes are detrimentally impacted by discriminatory policy decisions. To make meaningful improvements on the mental health of BIPOC youth, intentional decisions must be made to implement policies that promote healthy families and communities. Clinical work must be informed by an understanding of these structural and sociopolitical drivers of inequity, which begin long before patients step into a psychiatrist's office.

Trauma in BIPOC Communities and the Need for Trauma-Informed Care Settings

"Growing up, I had to go through gang violence and multiple forms of abuse, all while being a young man trying to figure out his identity and what it meant to navigate the world. I didn't feel like I had support from my family, teachers, or other adults in my life. It always felt safer and more practical to bottle up my emotions. Eventually I would find other ways to alleviate the stress of holding it all in, even if they were harmful."

Deleterious social determinants of health, created and perpetuated by structural racism, increase trauma exposures for many BIPOC youth. While initially an adaptive physiologic response to stressful situations,[17] stress pathways cause toxic stress when overactivated or prolonged, as seen in traumatic experiences.[18] Youth experiencing trauma are particularly vulnerable to toxic stress due to sensitive and critical periods of brain development in childhood and can consequently develop expressions of stress and trauma that clinicians have historically labeled as "abnormal," including emotional dysregulation, mood disorders, conduct disorder, oppositional defiant disorder (ODD), and disruptive mood dysregulation disorder.[19–21] Drawing from new neuroscientific information and conceptualization, trauma-informed perspectives recognize that youth exposed to chronic toxic stress must develop behavioral adaptations to survive their environment, a strength often not captured during clinical assessments.[18] To protect children and adolescents from academic expulsion, criminal activity, and legal involvement, we must ensure that trauma is appropriately and compassionately assessed, and appropriate resources are available for youth and families.[22–24] These trauma-informed approaches and practices are foundational to the success of any integrated care model.[25]

"I grew up in a mixed-status household where the concept of needing therapy was looked down upon because generations of people who had come to this country before me never had access to that kind of support. So, I'd get a 'ponte duro' (toughen up) before getting a 'talk to a therapist' from my own people and then be met with punitive responses to my behavior by school staff and other professionals."

Screening and prevention of trauma is a necessary foundational component of pediatric collaborative care models, as it is an effective, evidence-based, and cost-effective measure to improve not only mental health but also a broad range of health outcomes and quality of life indicators.[26] The Adverse Childhood Experiences (ACEs) Questionnaire is the most widely implemented tool for measuring the graded impact of trauma on physical health, mental health, and life outcomes.[26] As the initial ACE study surveyed mostly non-Hispanic White adults, further work remains to identify best practices for screening and support for BIPOC youth and families. One effort, the Philadelphia ACE Project, undertaken in predominantly Black inner city neighborhoods in Philadelphia, established additional ACE measures of residence in disenfranchised urban settings, neighborhood safety, bullying, witnessing violence, racism, and exposure to the foster care setting.[27] Importantly, the intersectionality of BIPOC youth must be considered when assessing for trauma, as they are more likely to experience a traumatic event not captured on standard trauma assessments, such as migration-related trauma, and are less likely to seek mental health care.[28–30]

As a teenager, I was constantly approached by different adults who would ask me questions about my life, or the experiences that I was going through, but the focus was always on the negatives, the struggles, the challenges. It was never about things that made me happy, helped me feel safe, or provided space for me to actually thrive. I remember constantly feeling like I was repeatedly having the same conversations with all the adults who I interacted with—teachers, counselors, doctors, and everyone else who saw that I was struggling. It might have looked like everyone wanted to help, but it sure seemed that nobody was talking to each other to make sure I felt supported and included in decisions about my life or mental well-being.

With the significant health-related consequences of childhood trauma, it is critical to identify trauma exposure early to prevent accumulation of toxic stress. As children traditionally do not reach psychiatric clinics until behaviors are externalized, collaborative models of screening and referral are imperative. One such model of state-wide screening was implemented by California in 2020. Under the ACEs Aware Initiative, spearheaded by California Surgeon General Nadine Burke Harris, state agencies partnered with research institutions to provide guidelines on the identification, assessment, and treatment of trauma in children, including the refinement of the ACEs questionnaire for pediatrics (Pediatric ACEs and Related Life-event Screener).[31] Screening can identify low, intermediate, or high risk of having toxic stress physiology, which then allows pediatricians to use comprehensive trauma-informed care plans to treat toxic stress or refer as needed.[32,33] The program emphasizes the importance of a network of care that includes collaboration between clinicians, community health workers, social workers, school agencies, and other community support resources to provide comprehensive support against the long-reaching consequences of trauma. Notably, many of the services provided under the ACES Aware Initiative are covered benefits through Medi-Cal, the California-administered Medicaid program.[34] With BIPOC youth experiencing disproportionate levels of trauma exposure during childhood, collaborative models such as the ACEs Aware Initiative provide cross-sector frameworks for preventing, screening for, and treating ACEs and toxic stress.

Centering Community in Collaboration

Increasing evidence demonstrates that integrated care models are an effective route to reach minoritized groups, with most of the studies reviewing outcomes for Black, Hispanic, and Asian-American patients.[35] A limited number of studies also indicate the effectiveness of collaborative care principles for Native American and Alaska Native patients.[36] The original collaborative care model is predicated on a highly medicalized model of disease and treatment, and in addition to appropriate linguistic services, some BIPOC communities may benefit from broader inclusion of culturally relevant figures or medical paradigms. Regular access to primary care services, a key component of the collaborative care model, may also be scarce in some BIPOC communities, whether in rural or urban areas, or on a reservation, and must be accounted for. It is important to note that while integrated care models may seem to be effective systems of care for BIPOC patients, their utility and success are also incumbent on centering community-relevant challenges, health beliefs, and practices.[37]

Diagnostic Presentations and Considerations

When people used to look at me, it felt that all they saw was a young, angry,gang-bangingalcoholic who needed to be arrested and locked up. Nobody saw the emotional trauma I had experienced or the pain that I was in. Everyone treated me like a criminal who also had "behavioral issues", not a young man who needed mental health support.

The fields of child development and child psychiatry have fluctuated in the understanding of normal and "abnormal" behavior. The understanding of what requires medical treatment, as opposed to nonmedical psychosocial interventions, continues to evolve. However, the current fee-for-service based medical model does not allow child psychiatrists to fully apply their extensive knowledge and understanding of the intersection between biology, psychology, and the social sciences to better assess and address patients' needs. Trauma-informed, culturally humble, and patient-centered practices necessitate questioning highly pathologizing labels and categorization of externalizing behaviors in children, especially those that may be better explained by neurodiversity, or trauma and stress responses.[18] In a recent call to revise diagnoses such as ODD, physicians from numerous specialties have described the intersection between stigmatizing diagnoses and how a child is treated by the adults entrusted with their care.[38] This subject is of especially high concern for BIPOC youth who, due to white supremacy and racism, are at elevated risk for pathologizing diagnoses and criminalization.[2,15,16,39]

WhenIwas26 year old, I was diagnosed with PTSD, Bipolar II disorder, and depression. At that point in my life, it was useful to have language and information to make sense of all the things I experienced as a child. However, if I had been labeled all of these things when I was young, many of the adults in my life would have immediately looked at and treated me differently. A young person will live up to the label and diagnoses we give them. People used to call me defiant and angry, and as a result I believed that I needed to act out in those ways. Many adults in my life also saw me that way. Mental health professionals can lead the way in usingstrength-basedlanguage when we talk about and support young people. When we give young people labels, they might internalize it for the rest of their lives. Not only that, but other adults and systems will automatically use those labels to treat them in a particular way that may not be what they need.

Children have a human right to safety, love, and wellbeing.[40] The "best interest of the child," the current standard for legal and medical decision-making, prioritizes the need of children for a safe and loving family with adequate psychosocial support.[41]

BIPOC youth and families, more commonly than their white counterparts, are separated, rather than supported, by the child welfare system.[42] Within psychiatry, child and family mental health systems have also deviated from these values. As psychodynamic and ecological assessment and treatments have often been replaced by manualized therapies and an over-reliance on medications, the application of holistic approaches to the treatment of externalizing behaviors in children has been diminished. Many child mental health clinicians encounter a disjointed approach to treatment whereby the child's externalizing behaviors are pathologized and often treated with medication, while the family and community mental health needs, such as interpersonal violence, use of corporal punishment, poverty, and housing instability, are not addressed in any purposeful manner.[43]

Any time I was offered support in school, from law enforcement, or any other public support, it was to put me on meds or throw me into a program where I felt like I had no control over my decisions or the environment I was in. The 'support' oftentimes never even really addressed the conditions at home or in my life that were leading to how I was feeling and acting.

To improve equity in child mental health systems, we must examine the language used to describe behavior, reassess which behaviors are pathologized, and reengage psychosocial and systemic interventions to protect children and families. Grassroots efforts have called to dismantle oppressive systems that have harmed BIPOC youth and families for decades; as physicians who took an oath to do no harm, we must use our voices and expertise to answer these calls to action.[44,45] Using collaborative care principles to center community, connect siloed systems, and increase access to trauma-informed interventions, offers a window of opportunity to accomplish some of these goals.

Traditional Collaborative Care Models

Psychiatric disorders in children are often initially diagnosed within primary care settings, and many children with mental health diagnoses do not receive counseling or treatment from mental health professionals.[46] Integrating psychiatric services into other child-focused sectors offer an opportunity to increase access to services for vulnerable populations and may aid in mitigating the disparities in mental health care access and outcomes. Integrating care is also more resource-efficient and less workforce intensive, as children are screened for need and many treatments can be provided without referrals to dedicated psychiatric clinics.[6,47]

Comparison of Select Integrated Care Models	
"Collaborative Care Model"	• On-site behavioral care managers • Psychiatric consultants (on- or off-site) • Record sharing • Outcomes driven
Behavioral Health Clinician Model	• On-site behavioral health clinician warm handoffs, shared records • Patients seen in real time • Optional record sharing
Child Psychiatry Access Program Model	• Off-site psychiatric consultants or therapists • Immediate consultation via telemedicine • No shared records • Primary aim of increasing geographic access to mental health care

Many integrated care models use one of the 3 traditional pathways. Perhaps most well-known is the collaborative care model, a "specific type of integrated care developed at the University of Washington that treats common mental health conditions such as depression and anxiety that require systematic follow-up due to their persistent nature."[48] This model uses on-site behavioral care managers and on- or off-site psychiatric consultants. This system is outcomes driven and records are shared between all clinicians and care managers. Another model is the behavioral health clinician model. This model allows for real-time collaboration by an on-site behavioral health clinician and includes warm handoffs and shared records.[49] Child Psychiatry Access Programs (CPAP), are "state-specific, publicly funded programs established to increase access to high-quality pediatric mental health care services by supporting primary clinicians in their role as mental health providers through telephone and occasional in-person clinical consultation."[50] CPAP's consist of off-site psychiatric consultants or therapists, and rely on telemedicine consultation to increase geographic access to mental health care. A limitation of this system is that telemedicine-based consultations may be less comprehensive and there are no shared records, making collaboration harder.[49] Though integrated care models vary, each shares the common goal of increasing access to psychiatric care for patients who may not otherwise be able to be seen in a traditional psychiatric clinic.

Expanding Collaborative Care Principles to the Community

Sometimes there were teachers and counselors I wanted to share with about what I was going through, but it always felt like they had very little patience for me. It felt like I was quickly dismissed as always acting out, maybe because I wasn't able to communicate well with them about what was happening at home. I needed more adults in my life trying to help me, but at the time I just felt ignored and like I had to figure everything out on my own.

Historically, integrated care often referred to coordination between a psychiatrist and primary care physician, whereby the psychiatrist operated as a consultant to the primary care physician who was the actual provisioner of services. However, many other professionals interface much more frequently with youth and their families than physicians, such as school nurses, teachers, social workers, and juvenile legal case managers. Using principles from collaborative care, they may be ideal partners in collaborating to support youth and their families.

Implementing integrated care models, not only in pediatric clinics but in other youth-serving sectors, is not new. Unfortunately, implementation is often met with many obstacles, and BIPOC children continue to be restricted from accessing care. By expanding care past the clinic, and into settings whereby vulnerable youth are most impacted, such as schools, juvenile legal, and child welfare systems, we might see progress in identifying high-risk BIPOC youth, increasing their access to treatment, and preventing future pathology (**Table 1**).

Using Collaborative Care Principles in the Educational System

The first time I was arrested, I was picked up off the street for not being in school and being intoxicated. All the officers did was ask me my age. Because I was young, they just shoved me into the police car and dropped me off at school without much conversation with anyone else. Then the dean came to lecture me about how what I was doing was wrong and that they would be telling my parents. Then I would get home, get yelled at, and because of how impulsive I was, I would just get even more angrier and just not want to be at home or school anymore. All adults did at that point of my life was lecture me or punish me. Where was the help?

Existing service gaps

Schools have been tasked with developing programs to address the social, emotional, and behavioral needs of their students and many offer some type of integrated school-based mental health (SBMH) services (eg, prevention; early identification; individual, group, or family counseling) through school- or district-based mental health providers, school health/mental health clinics, or through formal relationships with community mental health providers.[51] Schools have access to nearly the entire population of children and adolescents, which places them in a unique position to provide a range of interventions to prevent and treat youth mental health problems.[51] Systemic racism has resulted in policies, such as neighborhood redlining, that have resulted in inadequate funding to certain schools to provide equitable school-based mental health services. Many of the poorest districts in the US serve the highest concentration of Black students; these schools, in turn, receive far fewer resources than all other schools.[52] For K-12 grades; compared with White students, Black students are 3.2 times more likely to be suspended or expelled, Native American students are 2.0 times more likely, and Hispanic/Latinx students are 1.3 times more likely.[53] Even though suspension and expulsion have not been shown to decrease problematic behaviors or improve school achievement, these are the most common corrective interventions undertaken in education systems. Children with higher rates of mental health symptoms are not only at a greater risk for being subjected to exclusionary discipline practices, but also experience negative mental health effects because of detentions or suspensions. This bidirectional effect of exclusionary discipline increases psychological distress and emotional disturbances for BIPOC youth and contributes to the school-to-prison pipeline.[15] Schools have become a place whereby students, especially BIPOC students, are exposed to structural violence and then punished for displaying distress.[14]

Opportunities for collaborative interventions

While I was in prison, I met one teacher who started to see me as more than an angry,gang-banging,Latino young man. He saw me as a student, a young man capable of more. He helped me improve my writing, myself-confidence,and connected me to more people from my community who wanted to help me succeed upon my release. He connected me to other programs and professionals from different spaces. He was the first person to teach me that it was okay to ask for help, and the first time I experienced leaning on adults for support.

Implementation of collaborative care models in schools may support BIPOC students in the classroom instead of delegating services to the criminal legal system.[54] Key functions of collaborative roles in the school setting include initial identification of cases, assessment of needs with or without a diagnosis, liaising and coordination with service providers and recipients (including families), and psychosocial intervention delivery, among others.[51] If these are robust, reliance on pharmacologic interventions would lessen. Implementation of such a system would hinge on repurposing key players in school administrations. For example, with training, a school nurse, counselor, social worker, or school psychologist may be able to assume the role of care manager, and act as a liaison between the student in need of services, teachers, those providing interventions, and family. The success of such a collaborative model would require significant investments in care managers and wrap-around services. Otherwise, already overburdened school support staff will simply be given additional responsibilities without accompanying resources or support. Similar to how primary care clinic collaborative models demonstrated a

$6 gain for every $1 spent, preliminary evidence predicts that investment in student mental health, including BIPOC students, may also yield a positive return on investment.[55-57]

Collaborative Care Principles and the Juvenile Legal System

Existing service gaps

Systemic racism disproportionately exposes BIPOC communities to the criminal legal system, perpetuating trauma and incarceration for BIPOC youth. Beginning as early as preschool, these students are restricted from educational opportunities and exposed to carceral environments, often for minor infractions. One proposed initiative to reduce the school-to-prison pipeline is a minimum age for juvenile legal jurisdiction, with many stakeholders advocating for state and federal laws to set the minimum age of criminal responsibility at no younger than 12 years of age.[58] Other initiatives put forth include removing police from schools, abolishing zero tolerance policies, and referral to support services instead of arrest or prosecution—all of which require collaboration with community-based alternatives. Black children are more often incorrectly judged to be older and less innocent-appearing than peers, are misconceived as insubordinate and aggressive, and are therefore treated as though they require less comfort, support, and protection.[39]

Opportunities for collaborative interventions

Primary goals of collaborative interventions for BIPOC youth in the juvenile legal system should be to prevent exposure, and for youth already involved, extricate and prevent reentry.[59] For youth already in the legal system, effective collaboration can facilitate and monitor transitions from one system to another, facilitate the use of assessment information to match youth to appropriate programs, and promote active case management (eg, making or managing appointments, providing transportation) to improve treatment engagement and retention.[60,61] Foster and colleagues (2004) analyze the differences between 2 juvenile detention centers when the collaborative care principles are in place versus not. An example in Stark County, Ohio has integrated systems of care in the departments of program administration, financing, service delivery, and training for juvenile legal personnel from the mental health agency stationed at the facility. When compared with juvenile detention centers with similar demographics but without system integration, the likelihood of a youth committing a serious crime decreased by 57% compared with control sites (**Table 1**).[61]

Political Determinants of Mental Health for BIPOC Youth—Opportunities for Collaborative Progress

Policy change is needed to promote systems that can support the healthy development of all children and adolescents, including BIPOC youth, and to provide support and treatment when environmental factors or psychiatric symptoms impair them from being successful. Broadly, policies that address the sociopolitical determinants of health for BIPOC families and communities, such as access to health care and clinical crisis services, will have downstream benefits for the mental health of BIPOC youth. Additionally, policies specifically promoting collaboration and coordination of mental health care for BIPOC youth will also improve outcomes. Structurally competent clinicians able to educate policymakers on these measures will be instrumental in advocating for the systemic changes required to meaningfully improve outcomes.

A substantial body of literature documents the inability of biomedicine to meaningfully improve health outcomes in minoritized communities.[2,14,62] Often, these outcomes are mediated by structurally racist policies, such as those that limit the ability of BIPOC

Table 1
Windows of Access for Interception and Collaboration by Sector

General Pediatric clinic	• Traditional collaborative care models • Expanding the traditional collaborative care model to include other stakeholders • Accessible child psychiatry telehealth services • Trauma-informed screening • Increase trauma-informed care practices • Reduce focus on numbers and milestones, instead embrace a holistic approach to family care
Juvenile legal settings	• Diversion and "second chance" programs • Providing adequate psychiatric evaluation and treatment of detained children, including nonpharmacologic options • Linkage with postincarceration transition services
Community mental health clinic	• Trauma-informed screening • Increase number of BIPOC clinicians • Interprofessional collaboration with other sectors (education, legal, foster services & child welfare) to enable timely access for assessment, treatment, and support
Educational settings	• Qualified staff for screening for mental health needs • Accessible referral options • Age-appropriate mental health curriculum • Telehealth expansion • Wrap-around services • Remove/reduce police • Trauma informed and anti-racist educational practices • Remove zero-tolerance policies
Child welfare services	• Trauma-informed education for parents and caregivers • Incentivizing communication and collaboration between case workers and mental health clinicians (reimbursable services, "health passport")
Substance use treatment	• Integrated dual-diagnosis services along the entire continuum of care
Emergency Services	• Culturally and linguistically appropriate lifeline services (including texting line) • Child & adolescent mobile crisis services • Crisis stabilization units/Emergency screening units • Accessible wrap-around services • Services funded and provisioned through health agencies and community-based organizations instead of law enforcement
Trauma-informed Policy Interventions	• Clear, proactive and purposeful antiracism • Centering community-specific challenges and strengths • Perinatal health insurance coverage • Protected family leave (for both parents)

families to access health insurance and parental leave. As accessibility and affordability of health insurance is an important factor in promoting mental health, policies that increase coverage for not only BIPOC youth, but their parents as well, will also improve health outcomes among their children. Examples of policy targets to improve health care access for BIPOC youth and families includes removal of immigration-based limitations, coverage of prenatal and postpartum maternal care, and adequate funding of safety net hospitals and community health centers, including Indian Health Services programs. Accessible family leave is another policy target, as providing parents with the flexibility to care for themselves and their children when needed has been shown to improve health outcomes for children and parents alike.[63-65]

Mobile crisis services are increasingly being recognized as evidence-based models to effectively respond to mental health crises and reduce the overexposure of BIPOC communities to the public health threat of police violence.[66-68] Clinical crisis services provide an ideal intercept for individuals in crisis who may benefit from longitudinal psychiatric treatment or social support. Accessibility of mobile crisis response for BIPOC youth continues to be a challenge, as the prioritization of policing over investment in community services in minoritized neighborhoods continues in many areas.[2] The upcoming development of 988 as a nationwide mental health crisis calling code provides a singular opportunity for developing these services. Additionally, the ability of mental health clinicians to effectively provide and coordinate care for individuals in psychiatric distress will be required to decouple psychiatric emergency services from policing.[66]

Intentional policy decisions are also needed to incentivize, promote, and support collaborative models. Coordination and collaboration are requisite components for a system responsive to the needs of BIPOC youth. However, these services are often time-intensive and currently are poorly compensated, disincentivizing their implementation. Coverage models which account for the time and expertise required for collaboration of care, by reimbursing wrap-around services and social support, will help spur the development and utilization of these models.

Psychiatrists have important roles to play in collaborative settings, both as clinicians, as well as educating policymakers on the importance of data-driven policies for improving community health.[63] Structural competency and expertise to effectively

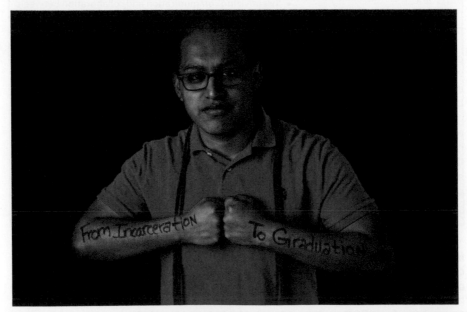

Fig. 2. The Journey of Hernán Carvente-Martinez: graduation from John Jay College of Criminal Justice, age 23.

coordinate across siloed sectors are distinct skills that can be learned during training.[62,69,70] Advocacy also continues to be an important skill lacking in psychiatry residency training, and should be emphasized as an important tool for psychiatric trainees and clinicians to improve the health of their patients and communities.[71]

SUMMARY

The current mental health system is not meeting the needs of our nation, including those of BIPOC youth. Contributing to this are national shortages of child and adolescent psychiatrists, underfunded child and family mental health-serving agencies, and most pertinent to this discussion, a severe shortage of BIPOC mental health clinicians. Worsening rates of psychiatric illness—including suicide—in BIPOC youth signify a need for new strategies among clinicians and policymakers. These strategies must account for the structural racism that overexposes BIPOC youth and their families to toxic environments, and concurrently restrict access to community-based support.

Mental health care models that emphasize collaboration and coordination with other child and youth systems present opportunities to provide targeted trauma prevention and mental health interventions for BIPOC youth who may not have access to traditional psychiatric treatment settings. These interventions should focus on supporting children, families, and the systems in which they live and learn. Pharmacotherapy alone is not sufficient and may lead to the overmedicalization of BIPOC youth. The development of these care models will open "windows of access" to care throughout the developmental timeline and can be implemented across various sectors. Combined, these efforts may improve outcomes and reduce overexposure of BIPOC youth to structural violence, including the school-to-prison pipeline.

Intentional policy decisions are needed to incentivize and support these systems, which typically rely on coordination and collaboration between clinicians and other supervisors and caretakers. Clinicians must be able to successfully navigate siloed systems and use their insight and experience to educate leaders on the importance of these policies. Advocacy continues to be a fundamental competency that clinicians must use for improving the health of their patients and communities.

As clinicians, it is imperative that we reexamine the harm we perpetuate through current diagnostic and treatment approaches, and we must listen to the individuals who receive our services to learn about these harms. Care and healing do not just include therapeutic interventions—integration and collaboration can and must occur beyond clinical settings. It is also imperative that clinicians recognize that healing and recovery can never be at the center of a system's mission, when the system, and the adults who work in that system, function to control, change and "fix" other human beings. Most importantly, as clinicians, we must remain humble and recognize that strength, beauty, and healing is already occurring within the communities we seek to serve. Our duty is not to save, change, or "fix" them—instead, we must support and walk alongside them, nurturing the strength that lies within. **Fig. 2.**

CONCLUSION

"I come from a background thinking that I wouldn't make it to 21, and that I wouldn't amount to much in life. So, I can't tell you the gratification that I get from helping even just one young person. Every success is a miracle and a huge accomplishment in my eyes."

Hernán Carvente-Martinez is a social entrepreneur advocating for prison abolition (**Fig 2**). His personal experiences with childhood trauma, mental illness, and incarceration compel him to advocate for pragmatic social change in the way we treat children, particularly Black, Latinx, Indigenous, and other children of color. Throughout this article, Hernán has shared history with wisdom and strength. He hopes that collaboration between community leaders, clinicians, researchers, legislators, and other stakeholders will occur to create sustained and meaningful progress.

DISCLOSURE

The authors have no conflicts of interest to disclose.

REFERENCES

1. National Healthcare Quality and Disparities Report. Services UDoHaH; 2019.
2. Bailey ZD, Feldman JM, Bassett MT. How structural racism works - racist policies as a root cause of U.S. Racial health Inequities. N Engl J Med 2021;384(8): 768–73. https://doi.org/10.1056/NEJMms2025396.
3. Services. USDoHaH. Youth risk behavior surveillance system. Available at: https://health.gov/healthypeople/objectives-and-data/data-sources-and-methods/data-sources/youth-risk-behavior-surveillance-system-yrbss. Accessed September 1, 2021.
4. Sheftall AH, Vakil F, Ruch DA, Boyd RC, Lindsey MA, Bridge JA. Black youth suicide: Investigation of current Trends and Precipitating Circumstances. J Am Acad Child Adolesc Psychiatry 2021. https://doi.org/10.1016/j.jaac.2021.08.021.
5. United States Census. United States Census Bureau. 2020. Available at: https://data.census.gov/cedsci/. Accessed September 1, 2021.
6. Asarnow JR, Rozenman M, Wiblin J, Zeltzer L. Integrated medical-behavioral care compared with Usual primary care for child and adolescent behavioral health: a Meta-analysis. JAMA Pediatr 2015;169(10):929–37. https://doi.org/10.1001/jamapediatrics.2015.1141.
7. Deo M. Why BIPOC Fails. Va L Rev 2021;107.
8. Sabshin M, Diesenhaus H, Wilkerson R. Dimensions of institutional racism in psychiatry. Am J Psychiatry 1970;127(6):787–93. https://doi.org/10.1176/ajp.127.6.787.
9. Wendel ML, Nation M, Williams M, et al. The structural violence of white supremacy: Addressing root causes to prevent youth violence. Arch Psychiatr Nurs 2021;35(1):127–8. https://doi.org/10.1016/j.apnu.2020.10.017.
10. Simons RL, Lei MK, Beach SRH, et al. Discrimination, segregation, and chronic inflammation: Testing the weathering explanation for the poor health of Black Americans. Dev Psychol 2018;54(10):1993–2006. https://doi.org/10.1037/dev0000511.
11. Williams DR, Collins C. Racial residential segregation: a fundamental cause of racial disparities in health. Public Health Rep 2001;116(5):404–16. https://doi.org/10.1093/phr/116.5.404.
12. Prevention. CfDCa. Racism and health. Available at: https://www.cdc.gov/healthequity/racism-disparities/index.html. Accessed September 1, 2021.
13. Jones CP. Levels of racism: a theoretic framework and a gardener's tale. Am J Public Health 2000;90(8):1212–5. https://doi.org/10.2105/ajph.90.8.1212.
14. Shim RS, Vinson SY. American Psychiatric Association Publishing. Social (in)justice and mental health. 1st edition. Washington, DC: American Psychiatric Association Publishing; 2021. p. 267, xxiv.
15. Fadus MC, Valadez EA, Bryant BE, et al. Racial disparities in Elementary school disciplinary actions: Findings from the ABCD study. J Am Acad Child Adolesc Psychiatry 2021;60(8):998–1009. https://doi.org/10.1016/j.jaac.2020.11.017.

16. Robles-Ramamurthy B, Coombs AA, Wilson W, Vinson SY. Black children and the Pressing need for Antiracism in child psychiatry. J Am Acad Child Adolesc Psychiatry 2021;60(4):432–4. https://doi.org/10.1016/j.jaac.2020.12.007.

17. Dhabhar FS. The short-term stress response - Mother nature's mechanism for enhancing protection and performance under conditions of threat, challenge, and opportunity. Front Neuroendocrinol 2018;49:175–92. https://doi.org/10.1016/j.yfrne.2018.03.004.

18. Trauma-Informed Care in Behavioral Health Services. Substance Abuse and Mental Health Services Administration; 2014.

19. Oakley C, Harris S, Fahy T, Murphy D, Picchioni M. Childhood adversity and conduct disorder: a developmental pathway to violence in schizophrenia. Schizophr Res 2016;172(1–3):54–9. https://doi.org/10.1016/j.schres.2016.01.047.

20. Ford JD, Racusin R, Daviss WB, et al. Trauma exposure among children with oppositional defiant disorder and attention deficit-hyperactivity disorder. J Consult Clin Psychol 1999;67(5):786–9. https://doi.org/10.1037/0022-006X.67.5.786.

21. Mroczkowski MM, McReynolds LS, Fisher P, Wasserman GA. Disruptive mood dysregulation disorder in juvenile justice. J Am Acad Psychiatry L 2018;46(3):329–38. https://doi.org/10.29158/JAAPL.003767-18.

22. Porche MV, Fortuna LR, Lin J, Alegria M. Childhood trauma and psychiatric disorders as correlates of school dropout in a national sample of young adults. Child Dev 2011;82(3):982–98. https://doi.org/10.1111/j 1467-8624 2010.01534.x.

23. Reavis JA, Looman J, Franco KA, Rojas B. Adverse childhood experiences and adult criminality: how long must we live before we possess our own lives? Perm J Spring 2013;17(2):44–8. https://doi.org/10.7812/TPP/12-072.

24. Marsiglio MC, Chronister KM, Gibson B, Leve LD. Examining the link between traumatic events and delinquency among juvenile delinquent girls: a longitudinal study. J Child Adolesc Trauma 2014;7(4):217–25. https://doi.org/10.1007/s40653-014-0029-5.

25. Brown JD, King MA, Wissow LS. The Central role of relationships with trauma-informed integrated care for children and youth. Acad Pediatr 2017;17(7S):S94–101. https://doi.org/10.1016/j.acap.2017.01.013.

26. Adverse childhood experiences (ACEs). Centers for disease control and prevention. Available at: https://www.cdc.gov/violenceprevention/aces/index.html. Accessed September 1, 2021.

27. Cronholm PF, Forke CM, Wade R, et al. Adverse childhood experiences: expanding the concept of adversity. Am J Prev Med 2015;49(3):354–61. https://doi.org/10.1016/j.amepre.2015.02.001.

28. de Arellano MA, Andrews AR 3rd, Reid-Quinones K, et al. Immigration trauma among hispanic youth: missed by trauma assessments and predictive of depression and PTSD symptoms. J Lat Psychol 2018;6(3):159–74. https://doi.org/10.1037/lat0000090.

29. The Trevor Project research Brief: Black LGBTQ youth mental health, 2020 Black LGBTQ youth mental health. 2020. Available at: https://www.thetrevorproject.org/wp-content/uploads/2020/02/Trevor-Project-Black-LGBTQ-Youth-Mental-Health-Brief_February-2020-1.pdf. Accessed September 1, 2021.

30. Elm JH, Dane, Abrahamson-Richards Teresa, Wall Melissa. Patterns of adverse childhood experiences and mental health outcomes among American Indians with type 2 diabetes. Child Abuse Negl 2021;122. https://doi.org/10.1016/j.chiabu.2021.105326.

31. ACEs aware. California department of health care services. Available at: https://www.acesaware.org/. Accessed September 1, 2021.

32. ACE screening clinical Workflows, ACEs and toxic stress risk assessment algorithm, and ACE-Associated health conditions: for pediatrics and adults. 2020. Available at: https://www.acesaware.org/wp-content/uploads/2019/12/ACE-Clinical-Workflows-Algorithms-and-ACE-Associated-Health-Conditions.pdf. Accessed September 1, 2021.

33. ACEs aware trauma-informed network of care Roadmap. 2021. Available at: https://www.acesaware.org/wp-content/uploads/2021/06/Aces-Aware-Network-of-Care-Roadmap.pdf. Accessed September 1, 2021.

34. Billing & Payment. California department of health care services. Available at: https://www.acesaware.org/learn-about-screening/billing-payment/. Accessed September 1, 2021.

35. Hu J, Wu T, Damodaran S, Tabb KM, Bauer A, Huang H. The effectiveness of collaborative care on depression outcomes for racial/ethnic minority populations in primary care: a systematic review. Psychosomatics - Dec 2020;61(6):632–44. https://doi.org/10.1016/j.psym.2020.03.007.

36. Bowen DJ, Powers DM, Russo J, et al. Implementing collaborative care to reduce depression for rural native American/Alaska native people. BMC Health Serv Res 2020;20(1):34. https://doi.org/10.1186/s12913-019-4875-6.

37. Lewis ME, Myhra LL. Integrated care with Indigenous populations: a systematic review of the literature. Am Indian Alsk Native Ment Health Res 2017;24(3):88–110. https://doi.org/10.5820/aian.2403.2017.88.

38. Beltran S, Sit L, Ginsburg KR. A call to revise the diagnosis of oppositional defiant disorder-diagnoses are for helping, not harming. JAMA Psychiatry 2021. https://doi.org/10.1001/jamapsychiatry.2021.2127.

39. Goff PA, Jackson MC, Di Leone BA, Culotta CM, DiTomasso NA. The essence of innocence: consequences of dehumanizing Black children. J Pers Soc Psychol 2014;106(4):526–45. https://doi.org/10.1037/a0035663.

40. Convention on the rights of the child. 2002. Available at: https://www.ohchr.org/EN/professionalinterest/pages/crc.aspx. Accessed September 1, 2021.

41. Carbone J. Legal applications of the "best interest of the child" standard: judicial rationalization or a measure of institutional competence? Pediatrics 2014;134(Suppl 2):S111–20. https://doi.org/10.1542/peds.2014-1394G.

42. Feely M, Bosk EA. That which is Essential has been made Invisible: the need to bring a structural risk perspective to reduce racial disproportionality in child welfare. Race Soc Probl 2021;1–14. https://doi.org/10.1007/s12552-021-09313-8.

43. Schut RA, Sorenson SB, Gelles RJ. Police response to violence and conflict between parents and their minor children. J Fam Violence 2020;35(2):117–29. https://doi.org/10.1007/s10896-019-00088-6.

44. Fitzgerald M. Rising voices for 'family power' seek to abolish the child welfare system. The imprint. July 8. Available at: https://imprintnews.org/child-welfare-2/family-power-seeks-abolish-cps-child-welfare/45141. Accessed September 1, 2021.

45. Roberts DE. Shattered bonds : the color of child welfare, x. New York: Basic Books; 2002. p. 341.

46. Whitney DG, Peterson MD. US national and state-level prevalence of mental health disorders and disparities of mental health care Use in children. JAMA Pediatr 2019;173(4):389–91. https://doi.org/10.1001/jamapediatrics.2018.5399.

47. de Voursney D, Huang LN. Meeting the mental health needs of children and youth through integrated care: a systems and policy perspective. Psychol Serv 2016; 13(1):77–91. https://doi.org/10.1037/ser0000045.
48. Collaborative care. University of Washington AIMS center. Available at: https:// aims.uw.edu/collaborative-care. Accessed September 1, 2021.
49. Dillon-Naftolin E, Margret CP, Russell D, French WP, Hilt RJ, Sarvet B. Implementing integrated care in pediatric mental health: principles, current models, and future directions. Focus (Am Psychiatr Publ) 2017;15(3):249–56. https://doi.org/ 10.1176/appi.focus.20170013.
50. Cama S, Knee A, Sarvet B. Impact of child psychiatry access programs on mental health care in pediatric primary care: measuring the parent experience. Psychiatr Serv 2020;71(1):43–8. https://doi.org/10.1176/appi.ps.201800324.
51. Lyon AR, Whitaker K, French WP, Richardson LP, Wasse JK, McCauley E. Collaborative care in schools: enhancing integration and impact in youth mental health. Adv Sch Ment Health Promot 2016;9(3–4):148–68. https://doi.org/10.1080/ 1754730X.2016.1215928.
52. National equity atlas. 2020. Available at: www.nationalequityatlas.org. Accessed September 1, 2021.
53. K-12 Education: Discipline Disparities for Black Students,Boys, and Students with Disabilities,. 2018.
54. Vandergoot M. Justice for young offenders. Needs, 2006 their needs, our responses. Vancouver(Canada): UBC Press; 2006.
55. Eisenberg D, Freed GL. Reassessing how society prioritizes the health of young people. Health Aff (Millwood) 2007;26(2):345–54. https://doi.org/10.1377/hlthaff. 26.2.345.
56. Eisenberg D, Raghavan R. Investments in children's mental health. New York: Oxford University Press; 2019.
57. Unutzer J, Katon WJ, Fan MY, et al. Long-term cost effects of collaborative care for late-life depression. Am J Manag Care 2008;14(2):95–100.
58. Tolliver DG, Bath E, Abrams LS, Barnert E. Addressing child mental health by creating a national minimum age for juvenile justice jurisdiction. J Am Acad Child Adolesc Psychiatry 2021. https://doi.org/10.1016/j.jaac.2021.02.019.
59. Owen MC, Wallace SB, Committee On A. Advocacy and collaborative health care for justice-involved youth. Pediatrics 2020;146(1). https://doi.org/10.1542/peds. 2020-1755.
60. Belenko S, Knight D, Wasserman GA, et al. The Juvenile Justice Behavioral Health Services Cascade: a new framework for measuring unmet substance use treatment services needs among adolescent offenders. J Subst Abuse Treat 2017;74:80–91. https://doi.org/10.1016/j.jsat.2016.12.012.
61. Foster EM, Qaseem A, Connor T. Can better mental health services reduce the risk of juvenile justice system involvement? Am J Public Health 2004;94(5): 859–65. https://doi.org/10.2105/ajph.94.5.859.
62. Metzl JM, Hansen H. Structural competency: theorizing a new medical engagement with stigma and inequality. Soc Sci Med 2014;103:126–33. https://doi.org/ 10.1016/j.socscimed.2013.06.032.
63. Bullinger LR. The effect of Paid family leave on infant and parental health in the United States. J Health Econ 2019;66:101–16. https://doi.org/10.1016/j. jhealeco.2019.05.006.
64. Aizer A, Currie J. The intergenerational transmission of inequality: maternal disadvantage and health at birth. Science 2014;344(6186):856–61. https://doi.org/10. 1126/science.1251872.

65. Baker M, Milligan K. National Bureau of Economic Research. Evidence from maternity leave expansions of the impact of maternal care on early child development. National Bureau of Economic Research. 2008. Available at: http://papers. nber.org/papers/w13826. Accessed September 1, 2021.

66. Rafla-Yuan E, Chhabra DK, Mensah MO. Decoupling crisis response from policing - a step toward equitable psychiatric emergency services. N Engl J Med 2021;384(18):1769–73. https://doi.org/10.1056/NEJMms2035710.

67. Jindal M, Mistry KB, Trent M, McRae A, Thornton RLJ. Police exposures and the health and well-being of Black youth in the US: a systematic review. JAMA Pediatr 2021. https://doi.org/10.1001/jamapediatrics.2021.2929.

68. Association APH. Addressing law enforcement violence as a public health issue. Available at: https://www.apha.org/policies-and-advocacy/public-health-policy-statements/policy-database/2019/01/29/law-enforcement-violence. Accessed September 1, 2021.

69. Hansen H, Braslow J, Rohrbaugh RM. From cultural to structural competency-training psychiatry residents to act on social determinants of health and institutional racism. JAMA Psychiatry 2018;75(2):117–8. https://doi.org/10.1001/jamapsychiatry.2017.3894.

70. Neff J, Holmes SM, Knight KR, et al. Structural competency: curriculum for medical students, residents, and interprofessional teams on the structural factors that produce health disparities. MedEdPORTAL 2020;16:10888. https://doi.org/10.15766/mep_2374-8265.10888.

71. Vance MC, Kennedy KG. Developing an advocacy curriculum: lessons learned from a national survey of psychiatric residency programs. Acad Psychiatry 2020;44(3):283–8. https://doi.org/10.1007/s40596-020-01179-z.

Parenting and Family-Based Care

Neha Sharma, DO, DFAACAP[a],*, Alexa Hooberman[b]

KEYWORDS

- Parenting • Racism • Acculturation • Mental health • Racial identity
- Family-based care

KEY POINTS

- Culture, race, and racism impact approaches to parenting and parental goals
- Parent-child dyad and families of color are negatively impacted by systemic racism, racial discrimination, poverty, and acculturative family distancing
- Through family-based care, providers can mitigate impact of racism and acculturative stress on parent-child dyad
- Cultural humility, curiosity, and respect are essential for successful family-based care

INTRODUCTION

In the current political sociocultural climate, there is a movement toward addressing systemic racism and disparate mental health treatment outcomes of youth of color. To address the mental health treatment outcomes of youth of color, one needs to provide family-based care that is culturally sensitive.[1] The provider needs to be accepting of the family values and the family goals. To truly appreciate families, their approach to parenting youth, especially in families of color, needs to be understood. In this section, we hope to review what parenting is, the sociocultural factors that impact parenting, and how one can provide family-based care to improve treatment outcomes of youth of color.

Background

What is parenting?

Parenting is a term that is used frequently but has numerous insinuations. It is absolutely essential to our being as put by Teti and colleagues, "Parenting is one of the most emotionally powerful, demanding, and consequential tasks of adult life. Long before modern societies emerged, extended family and community members shared

---

[a] Tufts Medical Center, 800 Washington Street Box 1007, Boston, MA 02111, USA; [b] Tufts University School of Medicine, 145 Harrison Avenue, Boston, MA 02111, USA
* Corresponding author.
E-mail address: nsharma@tuftsmedicalcenter.org

Child Adolesc Psychiatric Clin N Am 31 (2022) 313–326
https://doi.org/10.1016/j.chc.2022.01.003
1056-4993/22/© 2022 Elsevier Inc. All rights reserved.

childpsych.theclinics.com

the task of parenting. Today, without such a network of experience and support, it is a task for which we are often poorly prepared."[2] Without discussing parenting, one cannot consider providing family-based care. Anthropological perspective describes parenting as a means of socializing and teaching children how to interact with their environment to live and succeed.[3] More modern definitions of parenting refer to parents investing in their children's lives by providing resources that will allow their children to succeed.[3] This new definition developed in the context of rapidly changing values of one generation from the next due to technology. These "resources" that parents are expected to provide are influenced by what is available in their surrounding environment, cultural norms, financial security, access to knowledge of parenting, policies that allow supportive parenting, and systemic racism. Furthermore, the parents of racially and ethnically underrepresented youth also have the responsibility of supporting their children to navigate social messages that may undermine their wellbeing and go against their cultural values. When living in a different country or region where the larger community does not share the same beliefs, the pressure on parents to be the sole vehicle to transmit cultural knowledge and experience is accentuated, challenging the parent-child relationship.[4] Also, the definition of parenting always includes keeping youth safe; thus, families of color have an additional task when and if the mainstream culture views children of color as deviants and/or criminals.[5]

These two definitions of parenting are not mutually exclusive. Often parents' responsibilities are to support youth to socialize within the community while allocating the resources to set them up for success. This socialization is done through training, control, and a nurturing framework.[6] All these approaches are also influenced by culture and the cultural norms of the family. In cultures where mothers are responsible for food preparation—a proxy for not having the responsibility to provide financially as well—training to conduct increasingly complex tasks is the most common socialization approach. Control is a modality that is used to socialize youth in cultures where children have more free time because of chores being shared among a community. Control is exerted through threats, commands, and reprimands with limited explanations, such as in cultures like the Northern Indian and Tarong region of the Philippines.[6] A high controlling environment that has a negative, authoritarian, and punitive parenting approach is associated with increased psychopathology.[7] Nurturing focuses on encouragement, validation, and growth. In Western societies, control is used to socialize a child in a nurturing context.[6]

If the goal is to help the child socialize in "the world," a parent's perspective on that world and what "success" means in that world also influences parenting. In a collective society, a parent's goal would be to emphasize community harmony over individual growth. For example, in Japan, politeness is of large cultural value, so the child does not "cause trouble to other people."[6] In an individualistic society, individual growth is valued over community needs; thus, parents expect the child to "think for themselves" to be successful.[6] Furthermore, it is not just the culture of race and ethnicity but also the subculture of social class that impacts parenting. For example, parents in the American middle and upper class expect their children to solve complex problems, as if preparing them "to participate in a culture concerned with symbols and analytic problem solving."[6] Lower-class families socialize children to be obedient, polite, and conforming, likely to reduce adverse experiences for their children as often experienced by immigrant and BIPOC youth.[6]

Sociocultural Factors that Impact Parent-Child Relationship

Since youth learn and grow in the context of their family, anything that disrupts the family also impacts the parent-child relationship. Poverty is a powerful disruptor that impacts families and child development. According to the Children's Defense Fund, approximately 14.4% of children in the United States live in poverty.[8] This number is unfortunately higher in families of color, 20.5% of whom suffer from impoverished conditions. African American children have the highest poverty rate at 26.5%.[8] Poverty has been associated with poorer psychological health of the parents because of the added financial strains that make everyday life more difficult. Parents of lower income are also more likely to use punitive parenting techniques rather than reasoning and are less likely to display emotional affection. The burden of poverty cultivates an environment where parents do not have the time, attention, or patience for nurturing their child as much as they may desire[9]

With poverty decreasing the amount of time and/or money (for educational support), a parent is able to invest in the child's upbringing, parent-child relationships may go on to suffer more challenges than families of higher income. Low-income mothers with depression experience more conflict with their children than mothers of higher income.[10] Higher conflicts can be damaging to the parent-child relationship and lower quality parent-child dyad has been associated with poorer outcomes in terms of early cognitive functioning, relationship building, and self-regulation.[11] It is possible that the combined impact of poverty, sexism, and systemic racism results in limited bandwidth for parents to be fully present with their children while psychologically fighting existing microaggressive and macroaggressive experiences.[12]

DISCUSSION
Impact of Racism on Parent-Child Dyad

Parents of color and education
An important and greatly impactful aspect of child development is education. Schools as societal institutions are subject to influence by societal, cultural, and governmental structures that do not guarantee the inclusion of diverse families. Thus, the parents' interaction with school is also part of teaching socialization in a racist community while maintaining a sense of safety and educational and emotional nurturance for youth. From a historical perspective, the racist structure of schooling is well known; the classroom was a racially segregated space until 1954. School segregation was disbanded due to advocacy efforts by parents of color. Decades later, many educators still hold deficit-based beliefs about families who are culturally and linguistically different from their own.[13] In these settings, non-white parental behavior is often automatically associated with lower quality of parenting. In addition, the norms of parents' involvement in their child's education developed during the early to mid-20th century when white middle-class mothers were largely unemployed with ample free time to invest in their child's educational development. Thus, historically and currently, white parents are seen as "good parents" who work to serve the needs of the school while cooperating with educators. Meanwhile, parents of color, particularly low-income parents of color, are more likely to be perceived as being "inactive, disconnected, aggressive, or confrontational."[13]

Such bias against parents of color is unfair as parents of color often use other ways to be involved in their child's education. Parents of color remain engaged in both traditionally involved activities, such as reading with their children, helping with homework, and attending school events, while also engaging in community-oriented activities. Furthermore, they advocate for their children by negotiating with the predominantly white educational system and pursuing activism toward antiracist efforts. This activism, however, is often perceived by white educators as aggressive and confrontational.[13] The frequent notion that parents of color do not value education is invalid, as they perceive education as a means of upward mobility and encourage their children toward educational attainment. Unfortunately, "the efforts of women of color as fully engaged parents often go unrecognized and underestimated."[14] As one can imagine, if the parent is not feeling recognized by the school system, it would be challenging for the child to also feel valued. Furthermore, there are sufficient data to show that microaggressions by teachers and peers toward youth of color are a frequent occurrence.[13]

Parents of color and racism

Carrying the burden of navigating racist institutions, including the education system and beyond, parents of color address racism with their children through various methodologies. In fact, beyond overtly discussing racism, parents of color are constantly advocating for their children and protecting their children from discrimination while also modeling navigating systemic racism in everyday activities. Parents also experience the pressure of maintaining emotional regulation in unjust situations as the reaction of being angry is often out of proportion to the situation. They have to be mindful that developmentally appropriate mistakes and exploration, such as experimentation with clothing or substances, can be either sexualized or criminalized. Having experienced some of these traumatic experiences themselves, parents may have strong reactions that can stress the parent-child relationship.

Racial socialization profiles

Parenting in families of color may differ by the degree and manner of racial socialization, which refers to how parents discuss race and racism through both conversations and subliminal messaging. In an effort to better understand approaches to parenting in families of color, researchers have used racial socialization profiles to determine how a parenting style may differ depending on the gender of the child, discrimination experienced by the parent, and demographics such as family income (**Table 1**). In addition, racial socialization profiles have been used to understand associations between a certain approach to parenting in youth of color and outcomes such as resilience in the face of discrimination, racial identity, psychological well-being, and academic achievement. It is important to recognize that categorizing parents into profiles can cloud the more complex yet accurate view of parenting as a dynamic process over a lifetime. Therefore, such racial socialization profiles should not be viewed as fixed baskets into which parents always remain, but as small snapshots in a series of rich and dynamic interactions (see **Table 1**).

Psychological resilience was more commonly achieved when parents emphasized their culture, coping skills, positive messaging about race, and moderate bias preparation.[16,17,19] Overall, the combination of higher support and positive, culturally based racial socialization is associated with improved mental wellness of youth of color. Another dimension of support includes how involved parents are in the lives of their children; parents who are frequently engaging with their children are more likely to build resilience, refine social skills, and improve mental health in their children.[21]

Overall, experiencing racial discrimination was associated with poorer youth adjustment.[21] Racial discrimination was associated with increased depressive symptoms, increased perceived stress, and lower levels of overall mental wellness. However, a protective factor against these outcomes included parents who discussed race in a positive light.[19] In addition, experiencing racial discrimination as a parent was found to be associated with a multifaceted approach to parenting, where positive messaging and warnings about white environments were included in parenting.[20] This makes sense; mothers who are subject to combating racism are more likely to provide their

Table 1
Racial socialization profiles and significant findings

Study	Racial Socialization Profiles	Significant Findings:
Caughy et al,[15] 2011	• Silence about race • Cultural socialization emphasis • Coping emphasis/cultural socialization group • Balanced approach group • Cultural-supportive • Moderate bias preparation • High bias preparation	1. Male children are more likely to have parents who used the balanced approach and silence about race profiles. 2. Female children are more likely to have parents who use the cultural socialization emphasis profile. 3. Anxiety and depression were more common among balanced approach and cultural
Cooper et al,[16] 2015	• Infrequent racial socializers • Negative racial socializers • Positive racial socializers • Low race salience socializers • Race salience socializers	1. Male children are more likely to experience low race salience socialization than female children. 2. Female children are more likely to experience race salience socialization than male children.
Dunbar et al,[17] 2015	• Cultural-supportive • Moderate bias preparation • High bias preparation	1. High bias preparation is more common among mothers with male children. 2. Cultural-supportive profile and moderate bias preparation was associated with the least depressive symptoms in children.
Neblett et al,[18] 2008	• High positive • Moderate positive • Low frequency • Moderate negative	1. Children whose parents used the high positive racial socialization approach were less vulnerable to the negative impact of racial discrimination, whereas those in the moderate negative were even more vulnerable. 2. High positive approach was associated with best psychological adjustment outcomes. Low frequency and moderate negative approaches were associated with least favorable psychological adjustment.
Richardson et al,[19] 2015	• High discrimination/average parent • Average discrimination/average parent	1. Male children's parents more commonly fell into the category of high discrimination/average parent, whereas female

(continued on next page)

Table 1		
(continued)		
Study	**Racial Socialization Profiles**	**Significant Findings:**
	• Low discrimination/low parent • Low discrimination/high parent	children's parents most commonly fell into the category of low discrimination/high parent. 2. Male children whose parents had experienced high discrimination and female children whose parents had experienced average discrimination were more likely to be in the "detached" racial identity cluster in the 11th grade.
Smalls et al,[20] 2010	• Cultural affective-race salient • Low affective-nonsalient • Traditional affective-race salient	Children with the highest academic achievement had parents who used high racial messaging, child-centered parenting, and positive climate parenting.
Varner et al,[21] 2018	• Moderate positive (involved-vigilant) • Unengaged • High negative	1. Moderate positive (involved-vigilant) parenting is associated with youth resilience, competence, more refined social skills, and better mental health. 2. Best academic outcome was observed in moderate positive parenting. Least favorable academic outcome was associated with high negative parenting.
White-Johnson et al,[22] 2010	• Multifaceted • Low race salience • Unengaged	Mothers who endorsed messages that emphasize racial barriers to success had children who reported more frequent racial discrimination. Mothers who experienced more racial discrimination themselves more often used the multifaceted approach.

children with ways to protect themselves against such experiences. Knowing this information puts providers in a unique position to support parents of color to use skills that will make youth more resilient-positive racial identity, positive coping skills, and high engagement.

Academic achievement is greatest when children feel supported and are exposed to positive messages regarding their racial identity. Child-centered, high racial messaging parenting was associated with the best academic achievement, whereas parents who used minimal or negative racial socialization were more likely to have children with less favorable academic attainment.[21,22] Thus, for youth of color to thrive, racial socialization should be neither ignored nor viewed solely in a negative light. It is important for clinicians to encourage parents to assess what types of messaging they are providing their children with regarding their race.

How parents of color build racial identity

Aligning with the primary role of a parent to socialize children for success in their community, Manning discusses how black Americans seek out positive images of other black Americans to normalize black life for their children, including normalizing natural black hair, by viewing models in magazines or being members of black churches.[23] Black parents may also organize summer activities that expose their children to traditionally black activities, such as summer camps that are geared toward youths of color.[24] These camps provide a protected space where children do not have to justify their skin color; instead, they can feel safe to grow and learn about being part of their community.

Beyond encouraging children to involve themselves in black life, parents also teach their children how to navigate the world as they do. Black middle-class families may specifically seek out a predominantly white space to allow their children to observe how they conduct themselves in those spaces.[25] However, at the same time, understandably, some black families shy away from this type of immersion as they fear for their child's vulnerability to racial discrimination.[26]

African American parents often explicitly discuss race with their children to prepare them for racial discrimination they are unfortunately likely to face. Discussions include how to deal with police encounters, how to emasculate when confronted by an authority figure, emotional regulation, appearance, all of which are emphasized mostly in male children. In female children, the discussion centers around encouragement to join peer groups that celebrate black life and avoid media exposure that devalues black women.[23] Also, black parents encourage hesitation during interracial interactions as a technique to keep youth safe and promote black solidarity whenever possible to highlight racial identity.[23] The scientific literature about racial parenting is more focused on the experience of Black American families and less on the parenting of immigrant families. Below is a viewpoint that addresses immigrant families.

Barriers to Supporting a Child's Development: a Cultural Viewpoint

The ability to support a child's development is influenced not only by systemic inequities but also by cultural differences between the family and the society. Culture "defines what is right and wrong, what is acceptable and unacceptable for families, and what affects their everyday actions and interactions."[4] A family that is culturally different from the norm of their surroundings may have difficulty navigating spaces where the cultural expectations are dissonant. This can create barriers in a parents' goal of nurturing their child as a member of the minority community.

Acculturation is the change in values and beliefs that occurs when one is immersed in a different culture. The acculturative gap describes differences in values that may occur between each generation of family members. This may lead to acculturative family distancing (AFD), which is when the difference in values causes conflict within a family. There are two dimensions of AFD: communication challenges and incongruent cultural values. Difficulties in effective communication commonly arise from language barriers and differences in values.[27] Conflicts are brought about particularly when children enter adolescence and lean toward their peer groups as the primary influence of their behavior.

AFD can affect healthy child development as it can lead to hurtful family conflicts and rebellious behaviors which can cause the parents to be more controlling and rigid in their expectations. Owing to AFD, youth may not be able to use their parents for support during moments of stress, leaving them feeling isolated. This stress in turn negatively impacts a youth's identity, self-esteem, and mental health. AFD is associated with adjustment difficulties and increased symptoms of depression.[28,29]

Addressing Mental Health Outcome of Youth of Color: Family-Based Care

All the articles mentioned in this volume prove that mental health outcomes of youth of color are worse because of mental health stigma, systemic racism, and lack of resources that are culturally attuned. The increase in public health education, outreach to communities, and policy changes at institutions will address some of these factors. Many clinicians must still develop insight into the nuances involved in recognizing the dynamics needed to provide family-based care to mitigate disparities in the treatment of youth of color.

Families seek mental health treatment for a variety of reasons including challenges with the educational system, relational issues, behavioral issues, communication, and mood. For families of color, this connection with mental health treatment is additionally complicated due to mental health stigma, distrust secondary to historical systemic racism, and misclassification of cultural elements as inappropriate or pathologic. For example, often Muslim-American women who wear hijab anticipate being seen as "oppressed" by a provider. This engagement is more stressful when it takes place due to a mandate by a third agency; such as the school, legal, or welfare systems. Thus, the journey to a mental health provider has inbred distance and misalignment of goals that the provider needs to acknowledge and address to increase engagement.

The core tenets of providing family-based care is understanding that there is a 3-part system involved: the culture of the family receiving care, the culture of the provider, and the culture of the institution.[30] Furthermore, culture "influences how the members of the family communicate affection, support, and care and how gender roles and responsibilities are assigned."[4] Thus, in working with diverse families, it is imperative that the provider be willing to be a student of the family and the family's culture. Simultaneously, the provider has to be an expert in psychopathology and in the impact of mental health on development and life stages.[4] Remaining curious and respectful of the family and their experiences is essential to understanding their values and thus successful treatment.[4] The provider has to balance being aware of some of the cultural elements of the family's background while still recognizing that not all of the stereotypical cultural values will align with each family. This requires a balanced approach of openness, curiosity, and confirmation.

Family engagement with diverse families and evidence-based programs

Family-based care, when provided in culturally adapted programs, increases patient engagement, retention, and likely satisfaction. To understand cultural differences within any ethnic group, a historical perspective must be sought. In Africa, before slavery, strong men who acted as the providers and protectors were valued. However, this family structure was completely disrupted by slavery. Thus, patriarchy is less dominant in the African American family and family membership roles are considered more flexible than traditional white standards.[31] In addition, due to familial separation during slavery, African American families are more likely to rely on extended relatives for success. In contrast to the individualism that informs white American values, strong kinship bonds that cultivate a sense of community are emphasized in African American culture.[31]

Latin American families have generally historically immigrated to the United States in search of a better life for their families. Latin American culture values a stricter family structure where male family members are expected to be hard-working providers and female family members are expected to be compliant, caring nurturers.[6] Adults in the family often hold unquestionable power over youths.[32] In addition, Latin American families uphold the value of *familismo*, which represents a preference for closeness with family and a collectivist worldview.[33] Another crucial value that family therapists working with immigrant families should keep in mind is the respect for elders and parental authority, also known in Latino culture as *respeto*. Thus, Latin American youth in the United States may experience less flexible expectations for their role within the family than their white counterparts.

Asian American families generally value acting modestly, being considerate, regulating emotions, and self-sacrifice for the interest of others. Asian American families often reject the individualism that white American culture deems normative.[34] Asian American culture also endorses the patriarchal family structure and values caring for elders and educational attainment.[35] Mental health problems are seen as a familial issue that should not require outsider involvement; thus, contributing to mental health stigma and poor help-seeking behavior among Asian American youth.[35]

Over a 5-year study of African, Hispanic, Pacific Islander, American Indian, and Asian families, culturally specific versions of the Strengthening Families Program resulted in an average of 40% better recruitment and retention despite lack of improvement in the outcome. When there is a lack of an evidence-based program (EBP), it is best to identify evidence-based treatment for the patient then culturally adapt it. Cultural adaptation entails in-detail consideration of:

1. "Culture-relevant language, colloquialisms, and examples
2. Culturally accepted norms of role behavior
3. Culture-relevant definitions of undesirable behavior
4. Culturally and context-appropriate systems and service providers"[36]

The challenge of culturally modifying EBP is making sure you are not diminishing the foundational concepts of the EBP and not reducing the fidelity of the program.[36] With the increased usage of teletherapy and internet-based treatment, there is an opportunity to engage diverse families.[37]

Though there are not any randomized controlled trials of culturally attuned family therapy, experts in family work have written about it widely. For example, Boyd-Franklin wrote about working with African American families, and Bigner and Wetchler highlight means to engage with LGBTQ families.[38,39] Bernal and Domenech-Rodriguez made cultural adaptations to the Oregon Parent Management to engage with Hispanic families.[40] Attachment-Based Family Therapy when culturally aligned could be used to address parental guilt and worries about loss of cultural values.[41] In this approach, the provider works through relational reframe, alliance with the adolescence, alliance with the parents, repairing attachment, and promoting autonomy. To repair AFD, "practice of empathy and expression of overt support" is essential.[42]

Brief Structural/Strategic Family Therapy (BSFT) may be considered when working with African American and Hispanic high-risk youth.[43] There are 3 components of this model that include joining, family pattern diagnosis, and restructuring. Joining refers to the provider establishing connection, understanding their worldview, and collaborating with the family. Family pattern diagnosis is where the pattern of interactions that is causing or sustaining the problem is identified. Restructuring is the modification of these family interactions and roles of family members with the appropriate power structure accepted by the family. BSFT seems to be effective for African American families because it is present-focused and problem-oriented. By focusing on the present issues, BSFT can help parents develop ways of making their children more resilient against racial prejudice.[43] By being focused on the present issue and its causes rapport can be simultaneously built to eventually work toward past (distal) causes of the mental health problem including racism, psychological trauma, and social and economic injustice.[30] It is appropriate to acknowledge parents' worries about their child's safety and allow for a space to process these anxieties.[44] Finally, when working with black families, providers should encourage the development of a strong black identity in the youth to diminish the impact of racial discrimination.[44]

Addressing racism

Providers have not been good about asking about the impact of racism on the family. This may be due to lack of training on the topic, a collective sense of shame and guilt about our history, and discomfort in having difficult conversations. Avoidance only furthers the implicit bias, perpetuates the systemic racism in practice of psychiatry, and maintains the lack of cultural sensitivity when engaging diverse youth. Providers need to equip themselves with skills and confidence to have difficult conversations about racism. Ironically, this confidence in conversing about racism comes with the ability to acknowledge one's ignorance, mistakes, and desire to learn more. One way to develop this ability is to increase racism awareness and racial sensitivity. Lazzloffy and Hardy write that racial awareness is the "ability to recognize that race exists and shapes reality in inequitable and unjust ways."[1] Racial awareness can be increased by becoming familiar with the minority populations' historical journey and reading about its impact on day to day lives of that group. Racial sensitivity furthers racial awareness into action by anticipating how others may feel and think racially and accommodate actions appropriately. One example would be to understand how the practice of code-switching may be involved in the patient-provider interaction.

While remaining racially aware and sensitive, providers should engage in the "language of race"—being aware of direct and metaphorical racial comments. Providers must validate the experience of being racially targeted, dismissed, and oppressed and create a safe space for expressions of associated emotions.[1] A peer group or a supervisor to process emotional reactions and to highlight one's own bias and blind spots is valuable. Providers may also consider participating in an "ally" group that is focused on being antiracist. Simultaneously, it is important to be aware of the family's biases as well as the possibility of a negative perception of the medical field.[44]

When working with black families, it is important to keep in mind that not all families are the same. Inquire about the family's experience of injustice and systemic racism. Identifying themes of anger/rage, alienation, respect/disrespect, and the journey from boyhood to manhood can improve the level of therapy engagement. Meanwhile, African American male youth may become less engaged if issues of trust and mistrust are brought up.[45]

When engaging with all families, though more-so with families of color, it is imperative to bring up the potential impact of systemic racism and barriers on parents and youth. When specifically discussing racism, first speak to the parents about their views on racial issues and life experiences.[44] Identifying a parent's stance on the issue can guide future approach with the family. When family members disagree on the best ways to approach issues of racism, facilitate conversations, and remain nonjudgmental. These conversations have a reiterative process, often needing to be repeated with more understanding about the family in each cycle. Second, to address the problem of injustice and racism, focus on the changeable aspect of the problem.[1] Then, facilitate strategies to respond to racist remarks, control anger, and disengage when appropriate. Lastly, the provider must identify ways to advocate on behalf of the youth, including communicating with the school, the lawyers, and the medical team.

Addressing Acculturation Family Distancing

The degree of acculturation of a family has implications on the family system. When different family members are acculturating at variable levels, misunderstandings and communication challenges can develop. There can be different levels of acculturation in different dimensions of one individual's personality.[46] As per Sargent and Sharma, "Stigma around mental illness within the culture of origin, the degree of trust in mental health care, and a strong desire for a child's best outcome often influence the family's approach to treatment and their engagement in family therapy."[4] Thus, to address AFD, learning the family's way of understanding their challenges and honoring their language are the initial tenets to a successful treatment.

After grounding oneself in the narrative of the parents and the teen, the provider can develop mutual understanding and expectations to rebuild trust. The foundation is made stronger by reflecting resilient elements of the story or elaborating on the non-negotiable and recognition of love. This elaboration is pursued with a curious stance and humility that allows for development of meaning in the acculturative stress as well as trauma related to racism and postimmigration. With respect to the family's situation, reframing the challenges is easier. Family-based care is "a dialogue across four cultures, the culture of the parents, the culture of the child/adolescent, the therapist's culture, and the culture of mental health care. Navigating this dialogue is always a creative process that changes everyone involved."[4]

When the provider experiences countertransference or aligning oneself with the parent or the youth, believing in the parent's love for their child despite intensity of the expressed emotions can be grounding. Most importantly, "Understanding that this anger could be coming from a sense of parental failure is another powerful tool."[42] Often broader themes of concern shared by the parent and the youth need to be identified for further progress.

SUMMARY

In conclusion, parents have the single most profound impact on youth's development. Anything that impacts the parent-child dyad, including poverty, racism, discrimination, immigration, trauma, and acculturation differences, can modify the youth's trajectory. Thus, it is imperative that child and adolescent psychiatrists become comfortable in inquiring about the impact of racism, social injustice, and immigration on the family. They are in a unique position to facilitate a corrective process when equipped with skills to provide family-based care. The foundation of family-based care is humility, respect, and a curious stance.

CLINICS CARE POINTS

- Brief structural/strategic family therapy is a modified mode of family therapy that has been shown to be helpful in working with African American and Latin American high-risk youth
- Family-based care is essential to improving mental health outcomes of minority youth.

- Family-based care is integral in mitigating mental health impact of microaggression and macroaggression as well as acculturative stress.
- The core of family-based care is humility, respect, and acceptance.

DISCLOSURE

The authors have nothing to disclose.

REFERENCES

1. Laszloffy TA, Hardy KV. Uncommon strategies for a common problem: addressing racism in family therapy. Fam Process 2000;39(1):35–50.
2. Teti DM, Cole PM, Cabrera N, et al. Supporting parents: how Six Decades of parenting Research can inform policy and best practice. Soc Res Child Dev 2017;30(5).
3. Gadsden VL, Ford M, Breiner H. Parenting Matters: supporting parents of children Ages 0-8. Washington, DC: National Academies Press; 2016.
4. Sharma N, Sargent J. Family therapy with diverse families. In: Parekh R, Al-Mateen CS, Lisotto MJ, et al, editors. Cultural psychiatry with children, adolescents, and families. American Psychiatric Association Publishing; 2021. p. 233–48.
5. Smiley C, Fakunle D. From "brute" to "thug:" the demonization and criminalization of unarmed Black male victims in America. J Hum Behav Soc Environ 2016; 26(3–4):350–66.
6. Karniol R. Parenting and preference Management. In: Social development as preference Management: how Infants, children, and parents Get what they want from one another. Cambridge: Cambridge University Press; 2010. p. 89–106.
7. Wolfradt U, Hempel S, Miles JNV. Perceived parenting styles, Depersonalisation, anxiety, and coping behavior in adolescents. Pers Individ 2003;34(3):521–32.
8. The state of America's children 2021: child poverty. Children's Defense Fund. 2021. Available at: https://www.childrensdefense.org/state-of-americas-children/soac-2021-child-poverty/. Accessed October 10th 2021.
9. McLoyd VC. The impact of economic hardship on Black families and children: psychological distress, parenting, and socioemotional development. Child Dev 1990;61(2):311–46.
10. Lee C-YS, Lee J, August GJ. Financial stress, parental depressive symptoms, parenting practices, and Children's Externalizing problem behaviors: Underlying Processes. Fam Relat 2011;60:476–90.
11. Anderson RE. And still WE Rise: parent–child relationships, resilience, and school readiness in low-income Urban black families. J Fam Psychol 2018;32(1):60–70.
12. Nomaguchi K, House AN. Racial-ethnic disparities in Maternal parenting stress: the role of structural Disadvantages and parenting values. J Health Soc Behav 2013;54(3):386–404.
13. Chapman TK, Bhopal KK. Countering common-sense understandings of 'good parenting:' women of color advocating for their children. Race Ethn Educ 2013; 16(4):562–86.
14. Christianakis M. Parents as "help labor": Inner-city teachers' narratives of parent involvement. Teach Educ Q 2011;38(4):157–78.

15. Caughy MO, Nettles SM, Lima J. Profiles of racial socialization among African American parents: Correlates, context, and outcome. J Child Fam Stud 2011; 20(4):491–502.
16. Cooper SM, Smalls-Glover C, Neblett EW, et al. Racial socialization practices among African American fathers: a profile-oriented approach. Psychol Men Masc 2015;16(1):11–22.
17. Dunbar AS, Perry NB, Cavanaugh AM, et al. African American parents' racial and emotion socialization profiles and young adults' emotional adaptation. Cultur Divers Ethnic Minor Psychol 2015;21(3):409–19.
18. Neblett EW, White RL, Ford KR, et al. Patterns of racial socialization and psychological adjustment: can parental communications about race reduce the impact of racial discrimination? J Res Adolesc 2008;18(3):477–515.
19. Richardson BL, Macon TA, Mustafaa FN, et al. Associations of racial discrimination and parental discrimination coping messages with African American adolescent racial identity. J Youth Adolesc 2015;45(6):1301–17.
20. Smalls C. Effects of mothers' racial socialization and relationship quality on African American youth's school engagement: a profile approach. Cultur Divers Ethnic Minor Psychol 2010;16(4):476–84.
21. Varner FA, Hou Y, Hodzic T, et al. Racial discrimination experiences and African American youth adjustment: the role of parenting profiles based on racial socialization and involved-Vigilant parenting. Cultur Divers Ethnic Minor Psychol 2018; 24(2):173–86.
22. White-Johnson RL, Ford KR, Sellers RM. Parental racial socialization profiles: Association with demographic factors, racial discrimination, childhood socialization, and racial identity. Cultur Divers Ethnic Minor Psychol 2010;16(2):237–47.
23. Manning A. Racialized parenting in the United States. Sociol Compass 2021;15(8).
24. Butler-Sweet C. A healthy black identity" transracial adoption, middle-class families, and racial socialization. J Comp Fam Stud 2011;42:193–212.
25. Winkler EN. Learning race learning place: Shaping racial identities and ideas in African American childhoods. New Brunswick (NJ): Rutgers University Press; 2012.
26. Dow DM. Mothering while black: Boundaries and burdens of middle-class parenthood. Berkeley (CA): University of California Press; 2019.
27. Hwang W-C. Acculturative family distancing: Theory, Research, and clinical practice. Psychotherapy 2006;43(4):397–409.
28. Lane R, Miranda R. The Effects of familial acculturative stress and Hopelessness on Suicidal Ideation by immigration Status among College students. J Am Coll Health 2017;66(2):76–86.
29. Cano MA, Castillo LG, Castro Y, et al. Acculturative stress and depressive Symptomatology among Mexican and Mexican American students in the US: Examining associations with cultural Incongruity and Intragroup Marginalization. Int J Adv Couns 2013;36(2):136–49.
30. Mickel E. African centered family healing: an Alternative Paradigm. J Health Soc Policy 2002;16(1–2):185–93.
31. McCollum VJC. Evolution of the African American family personality: Considerations for family therapy. J Multi Couns Dev 1997;25(3):219–29.
32. Zafra J. The Use of structural family therapy with a Latino family: a Case study. J Syst Ther 2016;35:11–21.
33. Benson-Flórez G, Santiago-Rivera A, Nagy G. Culturally adapted behavioral Activation: a treatment approach for a Latino family. Clin Case Stud 2017;16(1):9–24.

34. Tsai-Chae AH, Nagata DK. Asian values and perceptions of intergenerational family conflict among Asian American students. Cultur Divers Ethnic Minor Psychol 2008;14(3):205–14.
35. Jacob J, Gray B, Johnson A. The Asian American family and mental health: implications for child health professionals. J Pediatr Health Care 2013;27(3):180–8.
36. Kumpfer KL. Cultural adaptations of evidence-based family Interventions to Strengthen families and improve children's developmental outcomes. Eur J Dev Psychol 2012;9(1):104–16.
37. Kumpfer KL, Magalhaes C, Xie J. Cultural adaptation and Implementation of evidence-based Interventions with diverse populations. Prev Sci 2017;18(6): 649–59.
38. Boyd-Franklin N. Black Families in Therapy: Understanding the African American Experience. Guiliford Press; 2006.
39. Bigner JJ & Wetchler JL. Handbook of LGBT-Affirmative Couple and Family Therapy. Routledge; 2012.
40. Bernal G & Domenech-Rodriguez MM. Cultural Adaptations: Tools for Evidence-Based Practice with Diverse Populations. American Psychological Association; 2012.
41. Ewing ES, Diamond G, Levy S. Attachment based family therapy for depressed and Suicidal adolescents: Theory, clinical model, and Empirical support. Attach Hum Dev 2015;17(2):136–56.
42. Sharma N, Shaligram D, Yoon GH. Engaging South Asian youth and families: a clinical review. Int J Soc Psychiatry 2020;66(6):584–92.
43. Tseng WS, Streltzer J. Cultural Competence in clinical psychiatry. Washington, DC: American Psychiatry Publishing Inc; 2004.
44. Kelly S, Jeremie-Brinke G, Chambers AL, et al. The black lives Matter movement: a Call to action for Couple and family therapists. Fam Process 2020;59(4): 1374–88.
45. Jackson-Gilfort A, Liddle HA, Tejeda MJ, et al. Facilitating engagement of African American male adolescents in family therapy: a cultural theme process study. J Black Psychol 2001;27(3):321–40.
46. Harper FG. With all My Relations: Counseling American Indians and Alaska Natives within a familial context. Fam J 2011;19(4):434–42.

Immigration and Race
A Challenge of Many Shades

Eugenio M. Rothe, MD[a],*, Arturo Sanchez-Lacay, MD[b]

KEYWORDS

- Race • Ethnicity • US racial topography • Racial-intermarriage • Discrimination
- Racism • Risk factors • Protective factors

KEY POINTS

- The article describes history of race relations and the present and future and the rapidly changing racial topography of the United States.
- It analyzes the complexity of ethnic-racial self-identification in the face of the increasing multiethnic and multiracial American population.
- It addresses the history of racism and discrimination experienced by minority populations and immigrants of color and the psychological effects of discrimination and racism on these populations.
- It describes the process of ethnic-racial identity development and the different styles of ethnic-racial socialization and cultural orientation. It describes the risk factors and protective factors that come into play when individuals are faced with experiences of discrimination and racism.
- It offers treatment recommendations on how to approach and discuss issues of ethnicity and race in psychotherapy in particular when treating immigrant and refugee patients.

INTRODUCTION

Migrations to seek economic or material improvement, or to move from a hostile and persecutory environment to a more generous and welcoming one, have been an important human activity throughout the course of history. The total number of immigrants in the United States is estimated at 40 million, and between 2000 and 2010 the United States received 14 million immigrants, the highest decade of immigration in the Nation's history. Latin America contributed the most immigrants, and Mexico was by far the top immigrant-sending country. Although the number of immigrants in the country is higher than at any time in American history, the immigrant share of the population (12.9%) was actually higher 90 years ago when a large wave of immigrants

[a] Herbert Wertheim College of Medicine/Florida International University, 2199 Ponce de Leon Boulevard, Suite 304, Coral Gables, FL 33149, USA; [b] BronxCare /Columbia University, BronxCare Hospital Center, 1276 Fulton Avenue, Bronx, NY 10456, USA
* Corresponding author.
E-mail address: erothe@fiu.edu

Child Adolesc Psychiatric Clin N Am 31 (2022) 327–342
https://doi.org/10.1016/j.chc.2022.01.004
1056-4993/22/© 2022 Elsevier Inc. All rights reserved.

arrived from Europe. Multiple factors influence migration decisions, but immigration is also driven, in part, by the social networks of family and friends that provide information to the future immigrant and facilitate their adaptation once they arrive in the receiving country.[1,2] Immigrant children and the children of immigrants also comprise an increasing proportion of America's younger population. Immigrants account for greater than 12.9% of the US population, but their children are greater than 23% of the population younger than 18 years, and about 2.2 million children in the United States are recent immigrants. Seventy-five percent of children of immigrants were born in the United States and are thus US citizens. Most of the children of immigrants—61% in 2003—live in families where one or more children are citizens but one or more parents are noncitizens. First-generation (children who were born outside the United States but immigrated) and second-generation immigrant children (children who were born in the United States and who have one or both parents who are immigrant) are the most rapidly growing segment of the US child population and account for greater than 30% of the US school population.[3]

The United States was once a country with a large white majority population and a small black minority with impenetrable color lines, but over the past 4 decades, immigration has increased the racial and ethnic diversity in the United States.[4] Along with increased immigration are increases in the rates of ethnic/racial intermarriage, which is transforming the American landscape into one with a growing multiracial population. Currently 1 in 40 persons identifies himself or herself as multiracial and this number could increase to 1 in 5 by the year 2050.[5] These demographic changes have occurred due to the arrival of unprecedented numbers of Latino and Asian immigrants, and new demarcation lines for race are beginning to develop.

DEFINING RACE AND IDENTITY

Race has been defined as a *"consciousness of status and identity based on ancestry and color"*[6] and *Identity* as *"the organization of self-understandings that define one's place in the world"* (p5).[7] Identity can be understood as a synthesis of personal, social, and cultural self-conceptions and has been divided into[1] *personal identity*, which refers to the goals, values, and beliefs that the individual adopts and holds,[2] *social identity*, which refers to the interaction between the personal identity and the group with which one identifies, and[3] *cultural identity*, which refers to the sense of solidarity with the ideas, attitudes, beliefs, and behaviors of the members of a particular cultural group. There is often confusion between the terms *cultural identity* and *ethnic identity*. *Ethnicity* refers to the cultural, racial, religious, and linguistic characteristics of a people,[8] and ethnic identity refers to the subjective meaning of one's ethnicity. Ethnic identity is contained within the broader concept of cultural identity, which refers to specific values, ideals, and beliefs belonging to the particular cultural group, and ethnic identity has always been a socially constructed product, which is affected by several variables.[9] Previously, Italian, Irish, and Eastern European Jews were regarded as *"nonwhite"* but were gradually accepted as white to distinguish them from blacks. After 1920, the cessation of the massive immigration from Europe that had begun a century earlier allowed these groups to no longer be seen as a threat to the American population. In the second part of the twentieth century, Hispanics and Asians began to migrate to the United States in large numbers. When asked to define themselves racially, more than 40% of Hispanics chose the *"some other race"* category compared with only 1% of the non-Hispanic population, in part because many Latinos see themselves as deriving from more than one racial group. In contrast, first-generation biracial Asian children are most likely to be identified as Asian compared with subsequent generations.[4] A study conducted among Asian biracial youth found that when asked to choose a single race, Asian-white youth are equally likely to identify as Asian or white, demonstrating that the racial identification of Asian-white multiracial youth is largely a matter of choice rather than a concept imposed by others. A second finding revealed that when a second language is spoken in the house, the children were more likely to identify as biracial.[10] The census reveals that whites account for 77% of the total US population, so most individuals who report a multiracial identity also claim that they have some White ancestry, yet multiracial identification remains uncommon among blacks. The Census Bureau estimates that at least 75% of the black population in the United States has multiracial ancestry (mostly white), yet only 4.2% of American blacks identify themselves as multiracial. The difference between black racial self-identification and that of the Irish, Italian, Jewish, Latino, and Asian immigrants, or descendant of immigrants, lies in the historical legacy of slavery, discrimination, and oppression to which black people have been subjected and which continues to marginalize this group, suggesting that racial classifications have a strong historical component based in racism.[10] The earlier studies on acculturation and adaptation to American society suggested that there was a single and unidirectional linear pathway to successfully assimilating into the nation's economic and social structure and that acculturation not only preceded but was necessary for incorporation into the structure of the host country. In this assimilation process model, immigrants lose their ethnic distinctiveness, become indistinguishable from the host society, and eventually adopt an American identity.[11] This model was applicable mostly to the white-northern-European immigrants who arrived in the United States before the 1920s. More recent studies[12,13] have proposed new concepts of *segmented assimilation*, with 3 possible pathways to incorporation into the United States: (1) a straight line assimilation into the white middle class (seen, for example, among light-skinned Cubans in Miami); (2) assimilation into the minority underclass (seen among the Haitians in Miami); or (3) selective assimilation, by which immigrants remain immersed in the ethnic community and preserve the immigrant community's values and solidarity as a means to achieve upward mobility (eg, among Punjabi Sikh Indians in Northern California).[5] Many of today's new Asian and Latino immigrants adopt a path of *"selective acculturation."*[12]

BLACK CARIBBEAN AND BLACK AFRICAN IMMIGRANTS

Black immigrants in the United States today number 3.8 million, more than 4 times the number in 1980, according to a Pew Research Center analysis of US Census Bureau data. Black immigrants now account for 8.7% of the nation's black population, nearly triple their share in 1980.[14] During the period of slavery, there was limited migration of black slaves from the Caribbean to the United States. Between 1920 and 1950 the number of Caribbean immigrants increased by 540%. The immigration reforms brought by the Immigration and Nationality Act of 1965 lifted the quotas of immigrants by national origin and replaced them with a system based on family reunification and employment, which further increased the number of Caribbean immigrants.[15] In addition, African immigration to the United States increased by 137%, from 574,000 to 1.4 million, and Africans now make up 36% of the total foreign-born black population. The largest numbers come from Nigeria and Ethiopia, who often arrive with substantial social capital in terms of higher educational including high school and college degrees attainment than the native Black American population. The same is true for Caribbean blacks, who have been portrayed as a "a highly successful model minority"; however, similar to African Black immigrants, levels of education vary according to country of origin. In terms of refugee status, most asylees were from Cuba (91%) and Haiti (9%).[16,17] This increase followed the de-colonization of many African countries in the decade of the 1970's and the larges numbers come from Nigeria and Ethiopia etc. Many black immigrants are from Spanish-speaking countries such as Dominican Republic, Cuba, Panama, and Mexico. In terms of levels of education, immigrants from Trinidad and Jamaica are the most educated, and those from the Dominican Republic the least educated.[15] However, once Dominicans arrive in the United States, their children make great strides in education taking advantage of the excellent New York Public school system, the city where Dominicans have established their ethnic enclave.[4] Many parents from the Caribbean immigrate alone, leaving children in the care of relatives back on the islands, and there is a significant amount of return migrations and shuttle migrations between the islands and the mainland, which causes parenting discontinuities and renders these children and adolescents vulnerable to mental health issues such as conduct problems, substance abuse, and poor schooling outcomes. However, among Afro-Caribbean and African immigrants, extended family arrangements are more common than among US natives, and this can be protective.[15]

EAST INDIAN, PAKISTANI, AND FILIPINO IMMIGRANTS

East-Indians represent the largest source of new immigrants to America, surpassing the Mexicans and the Chinese, and currently 4.5 million Indians or their descendants live in the United States. East Indian-American households have the single highest income level of any group in the country, more than twice as high as the general US population and only 6.5% of East Indian-American households live below the poverty line. East Indians arrived in 3 migratory waves. The first one occurred around the establishment of the Nationality Act of 1965. They were a selection of highly trained and well-educated immigrants; doctors, engineers, and scientists were overrepresented. Another cohort arrived in the 1980s as a result of family immigration quotas, and a more recent immigration around 2013 came with H-1B visas given to immigrants with specialized skills in professions that are in shortage in the United States. For this reason, East Indians remain a highly educated and financially successful immigrant group that skipped the "ghetto stage" of many early US arrivals. As a result of their British colonial past, most East-Indian families already speak English as a second language when they arrive in the United States, 92% have intact marriages, and they come from a country with a Democracy, offering advantages related to adaptation.[18] In spite of these advantages, many East-Indians experience discrimination and find obstacles for employment and full participation in American life.[19]

Filipino-Americans number approximately 4.1 million; about 32.6% do not speak English fluently and are the least likely group to seek mental health services, 3 times less likely than the mainstream US population.[20] Filipinos have a 400-year long colonial history by Spain and are overwhelmingly Catholic. They have a heavy burden of mental health problems, including depression, suicidal ideation, substance abuse, adolescent pregnancy, and human immunodeficiency virus.[21–23] Because of their long history of colonization, traditional Filipino immigrants tend to be fatalistic and have a degree of cultural mistrust of outside institutions that sometimes interferes with accessing mental health services. Catholic religion plays a central role in the immigrant Filipino culture, parents adhere to strict traditional values, they tend to enforce harsh discipline on their children, and problems are addressed within the family unit. Mental health services for Filipino-Americans have been found to be effective when they address (1) the intergenerational gap between parents and children, (2) when they collaborate with churches, (3) when they also address the parents' mental health issues, and (4) when they are evidence based.[20,21]

THE ROLE OF INTERMARRIAGE

In the beginning of the twentieth century intermarriage between whites and other groups was very rare, but today whites intermarry at such high rates that only 1 in 5 whites has a spouse with an identical racial–ethnic background.[18,19] Today, 13% of American marriages involve persons of different races, a considerable increase over the past three and a half decades, and the growth of the multiracial population provides a new reflection on the nation's changing racial boundaries.[24] However, this seeming erosion of racial boundaries does not include all racial groups. For instance, about 30% of married native-born Asians and Latinos have a spouse of a different racial background, mostly white. In contrast, only one-tenth of young blacks married someone of a different racial background and only 5.8% of blacks married whites. By contrast, the lower rates of intermarriage among blacks suggest that racial boundaries continue to be more prominent between whites and blacks.[25] In spite of the fact that the US Census Bureau estimates that at least three-quarters of the black population in the United States is ancestrally multiracial, mostly white, just greater than 4% of blacks claim to be biracial.[26,27] What sets Latinos and Asians apart is that their experiences are not rooted in the same historical legacy of slavery, with its systematic and persistent patterns of legal and institutional discrimination and inequality that have existed in the United States since the first slaves were brought to America from Africa. Unlike African Americans who were forcefully brought to this country as slaves, today's Latino and Asian newcomers are voluntary migrants, and consequently their experiences are distinct from those of African Americans.[4,5] The increases in intermarriage and the growth of the multiracial population reflect a blending of races and the fading of color lines and perhaps a reduction in social distance and racial prejudice, these patterns appear to offer an optimistic portrait of weakening racial boundaries. Yet, the continuing black-nonblack divide could be a disastrous outcome for many African Americans, who continue to incur extreme disadvantage due to segregation and structural inequalities.[4,5]

BIRACIAL IDENTITIES

Adolescence may be a stressful time for many youth in Western cultures, because it involves establishing a unique identity while also navigating peer group norms and societal expectations. Multiracial adolescents may face a more difficult challenge than their monoracial peers in that they must develop this new identity and decide how, or even if, they can reflect positive aspects of all heritages while simultaneously rejecting certain societal expectations and stereotypes.[28] A multiracial or multiethnic heritage can further complicate this process. By adolescence, most multiracial children have been made aware of any racial–ethnic differences between classmates and themselves. Often they are reminded of these differences as they attend school and are asked isolating questions such as, *"what are you?"* from classmates puzzled or threatened by their racially or ethnically mixed appearance. These alienating questions often contribute to the feeling that no one understands them, not even their monoracial parents. Concerns about "not fitting in" are magnified if multiracial adolescents discover that they are no longer welcome in certain peer groups because of racial issues. In addition, some peers, and even their own parents, may pressure the adolescent to identify with only one ethnic background, prompting feelings of guilt or disloyalty. Biracial youth oftentimes find themselves in a bind where they can either adopt the label that society gives them; choose to identify with both racial groups or only one of those groups; or choose to be known as multiethnic (or perhaps choose another racial group altogether). The therapist should stress that the decision is the youth's alone and that parents should be consulted but cannot make this decision for the child, and in addition, that the decision need not be made immediately and that it is acceptable to change one's mind later.[4]

In the case of children and families with biracial identities, a comprehensive review of parenting practices revealed that there are 3 main principles that can lead to the most culturally effective parenting[29] and these include the following:

Multicultural or racial awareness: knowledge of how the variables of race, ethnicity culture, language, and related power status operate in one's own and other's lives, including an understanding of the dynamics of racism, oppression, and other forms of discrimination.

Multicultural planning: if the family is involved in other groups, such as neighborhoods, schools, and churches that are exclusively or primarily made up of European Americans, the biracial child has no access to others like him or herself. Active pursuit of opportunities for biracial children to have access to other children of their other ethnicity or to multicultural can help normalize the experience of not being a member of the white dominant culture. This is particularly important for transracially adopted children, who should be provided the opportunity to learn about and participate in their culture of birth.

Survival skills: the recognition of the need for parents to prepare their children to cope successfully with racism. This skill is as important for children who belong to an ethnic and racial minority group, for biracial children, but especially important for transracial adoptees. For children in this latter group it may be more difficult to learn from European-American parents who have had little experience of racism directed toward them. Minimizing or ignoring racial incidents is insufficient for children who may find themselves at the receiving end of racially based prejudice or discrimination. These children need help to develop a strong self-image despite racism.[29]

LANGUAGE AND THE AMERICAN IDENTITY

Acquisition of unaccented English language has been, and continues to be, the litmus test of citizenship in the United States. In no other country are languages extinguished with such speed. To speak *English only* is a prerequisite for social acceptance and integration, and those who try to educate their children in their mother tongue confront immense pressure for social conformity from peers, teachers, and the media.[30,31] Several empirical studies highlight the fact that the *first generation* learns enough English to survive economically, the *second generation* (born in the United States to immigrant parents) may use the parental tongue at home but uses English in school, and in the *third generation* the home language and mother tongue shift to English.[30] Language use can also have subtle connotations in everyday life in America. Speaking "*accented English*," even by a native English speaker, can serve to highlight socioeconomic and cultural differences that can separate the adolescent from particular peer groups. A study conducted among first- and second-generation blacks in New York City noted that middle-class blacks convey, with mainstream English, verbal and nonverbal cues that they are not from the ghetto and that they disapprove ghetto specific behavior.[32] Also, oftentimes immigrant children growing up in impoverished communities receive no encouragement to retain their parent's native language, as the native language is stigmatized as a symbol of lower status[30]; this is very much the case for second-generation Haitian youth from working-class parents in Miami, who rapidly shed Haitian-Creole for English and prefer to be identified as *"American,"* rather than *"Haitian-American."* Yet, other studies involving language utilization in Miami, Florida found that Spanish was *"alive and well"* among first-generation Cuban immigrants but that language retention decreased in proportion to the length of stay in the United States. They found that in spite of the economic prosperity, excellent self-esteem, and social support offered by the Cuban *"Ethnic Enclave"* in Miami, 90% of second-generation Cubans preferred to communicate in English.[33]

DISCRIMINATION, RACISM, AND PERCEIVED RACISM AMONG IMMIGRANT YOUTH

As previously mentioned, projected population trends in the United States indicate that the country is becoming less white, with the share of non-Hispanic single-race white population expected to decrease from 66% of the population in 2008– to 46% of the population by 2050.[34] In spite of this, large-scale studies indicate that 87% of African American adolescents[35] and 50% of Latinos aged 18 to 24 years[36] have experienced discrimination in the past year and that these experiences of discrimination can have psychologically detrimental effects on some of these youth. There is substantial evidence of discrimination based on skin color for documented immigrants in the United States, with immigrants with the lightest skin color earning more than comparable immigrants with the darkest skin color. Current population trends in combination with an increasingly multiracial population is causing that the hierarchy of racial groupings traditionally perceived in the United States may be replaced by a hierarchy based on the skin color, in which persons with lighter skin color have an advantage relative to those with darker skin color, regardless of nominal race. In addition, this research also suggests that racial stratification in the United States is moving away from the current biracial system to one more as Latin America, with 3 racial strata that are closely related to skin color and that the darker a person's skin color, the lower he or she is likely to be on any scale perceived to be desirable in the United States.[37,38] The residual of the slavery and postslavery discriminatory laws and policies in the United States remains for more than 2 centuries after the abolition of slavery in the cultural portrayals that depict Black Americans with well-known negative stereotypes, including the standards of physical attractiveness that are based on European standards; thus, African Americans with lighter skin are viewed as more attractive.[39] Younger African American children tend to respond to the socially imposed stereotypes that lighter skinned black people are more desirable; however, once African American children reach adolescence, increased awareness of race and racial discrimination might foster pride in black skin, or alternatively, might lead to preferences for lighter skin because of awareness of white privilege. The attractiveness placed on skin color may also have variations by gender. A recent study found that lightness of skin tone for women was more valued, yet for men the link between skin tone and attractiveness was much weaker and not significant. Dark-skinned men rated themselves as more sexually attractive than fair-skinned men, suggesting that for men, dark skin may be perceived as an asset in terms of attractiveness. In contrast, light-skinned black women were more likely to be described as attractive and intelligent. The gendered nature of *skin tone bias* is also evident in the beauty products marketed to women of color, of which many are geared toward making women look more phenotypically white-skinned.[40] Hispanic newcomers, including many who are dark-skinned, poor, and undocumented, have come to perceive the social distance separating themselves from whites as more permeable than that separating themselves from blacks, and sometimes engage in distancing strategies to reinforce this distinction, but in many rural areas, the binary separation between blacks and whites remains strong.[41] For Hispanics, many of whom are biracial or triracial, the assimilation into the American mainstream, 3 possible outcomes can take place: (1) some Hispanics are allowed to "*become whites*" and are fully incorporated and assimilated (such as most of the Cubans in South Florida), (2) others are assigned to an intermediate group as "*honorary whites*," (3) and a third group are assigned to the group of "*collective blacks.*" Although some Hispanics may become "*whites*" or "*honorary whites*" due to their phenotype or higher socioeconomic status, most Mexicans, Puerto Ricans, Dominicans, and Central Americans are "*collective blacks*" due to their racialized incorporation as colonial subjects, refugees from wars, or illegal undocumented migrant workers. Still, some evidence points to a black-nonblack divide.[42]

RISK FACTORS AND PROTECTIVE FACTORS IN EXPERIENCES OF DISCRIMINATION AND RACISM

Racism can be conceptualized as existing in 3 levels: *institutionalized, personally mediated, and internalized*, and these 3 categories of racism are considered to be additive and synergistic.[43] An emerging research suggests that both perceptions of discrimination and internalized racism (endorsement of negative stereotypes of one's racial group) are associated with poor mental health. For example, studies have found that *everyday discrimination*, a form of modern racism that is subtle and ambiguous, is associated with increased risk of past-year major depressive disorder.[44] This finding is consistent with theoretic formulations of *interpersonally mediated racism* as a psychosocial stressor that increases risk of depression for people of color.[43] Experiences of discrimination and racism have also been associated with other adverse outcomes such as low self-esteem, poor life satisfaction, hypertension, increased risk of cardiovascular disease, obesity, and shorter leukocyte telomere length (a biological marker of systemic aging), among others.[45]

The particular impact of health and experience of Afro-Caribbean individuals provides an interesting example. Afro-Caribbean persons in the United States have been typically regarded as "*model minorities*". Previous research has shown that Afro-Caribbean persons in the United States have, in general, higher levels of socioeconomic standing, including education and income, and are also partly comprised of immigrant persons; all of these are known to be protective factors against poor mental health.[46] Paradoxically, some studies have found that Afro-Caribbean adults report higher prevalence rates of lifetime depression and depressive symptoms when compared with African Americans. However, the effects of discrimination on mental health seem to affect these 2 groups in similar ways.[32] Paradoxically, the *National Survey of American Life* found that among Afro-Caribbean respondents, but not African Americans, higher levels of internalized racism were associated with *decreased risk* of past-year major depressive disorder.[45] These findings were counterintuitive but similar to previous research that showed that by acknowledging the stigma that is attached to one's ethnic group, the individual uses the stigma as a point of departure and defensively distances himself from the assigned stigma in a self-protective strategy. In addition, *anticipatory vigilance*, a coping strategy that is characterized by monitoring and modifying one's behavior in an attempt to protect the self from anticipated racist events, can also serve as an effective defensive strategy to avoid the negative effects of racism. These investigators highlight the complexity of analyzing this data and the risk of oversimplification, concluding that just as the black population does not form a monolithic entity, the Afro-Caribbean group does not either, and that the decontextualized portrayals of black persons in the United States (immigrants and nonimmigrants) may conceal important similarities as well as variations across cultural, demographic, geographic, and social dimensions. Similarly, unauthorized Hispanics and other immigrants not only face challenges associated with being a minority in the United States, but they also face the additional burden of being an unauthorized immigrant, and they have been portrayed in the media as unwelcome burdens in US society. Together, these intersecting identities may exacerbate the perceived discriminatory experiences faced by this population. A study focusing on the risk factors and protective factors that mediated the negative effects of racism[47] concluded that *ethnic discrimination* is a salient stressor for unauthorized Hispanic immigrants but that a *high ethnic-racial group identity centrality* may protect these individuals from the negative effects of discrimination by providing a sense of belonging, acceptance, and social support in the face of rejection. When faced with discrimination, minority individuals can protect their well-being by increasingly identifying with their in-group, which may explain why ethnic identification tends to increase, rather than deteriorate, when individuals experience discrimination against their ethnic group. So, it is not mere ethnic-group membership that confers these benefits, but whether one's ethnic-racial group identity is *psychologically internalized* to form a central part of their self-definition and provide life with meaning. This is what is known as *ethnic-racial group-identity-centrality*. Such internalization of group membership is important because (1) it provides a cognitive framework for understanding oneself and one's place in the world. Also, (2) group membership provides a common perspective on social reality and furnishes individuals with increased feelings of belonging and purpose, providing them a better sense of control over their lives and more coping resources in the face of rejection, such as sense of social support and acceptance, and finally, individuals with high ethnic-racial group-identity-centrality may be protected from the adverse effects of discrimination,[47] (3) because they perceive their in-group as not deserving such mistreatment, which has been also found among minority groups such as African Americans.[48] In essence, empirical research has found that individuals with *high group-identity-centrality* report greater well-being as indicated by (1) increased personal self-esteem and life satisfaction, (2) decreased depressive symptoms, and (3) improved cognitive health. In contrast, members with weak connections to the ethnic group will experience more adverse effects of discrimination, because they lack a sense of social support, belongingness, and acceptance.[47] It is important to note that there are significant differences between first- and second-generation immigrants in terms of how each group values the opinions of others. So, for second-generation (born and raised in the United States with at least one foreign born parent) immigrants and for immigrants of color in particular, if they perceive that the white majority group evaluates their group less than positively, they are at risk if they do not have a strong connection to their heritage group or their parents' heritage group. In turn, if they have a strong connection to their heritage group, they can decide to ignore the views of the majority-culture group as bases for their own regard and pay more attention to the opinions provided by their heritage group. If they think that people in the heritage culture evaluate their ethnic group in the United States positively, they also evaluate it positively themselves.[49]

RACIAL AND ETHNIC IDENTITY, ETHNIC-RACIAL SOCIALIZATION, AND CULTURAL ORIENTATION

Racial and ethnic identity refers to the youth's attitudes and behaviors that define the significance and meaning of race and ethnicity in their lives. Positive identification with one's racial and ethnic identity seems to confer protection in several ways: (1) it may help to bolster self-esteem against some of the demeaning messages that are inherent in racial and ethnic discrimination experiences. (2) Racial and ethnic identity may make youth who experience discrimination less likely to make personal attributions (self-blame) for instances of discrimination, attributing discrimination to others instead, and thereby less likely to suffer from damage to their self-concept. (3) The effects of racial and ethnic identity on youth adjustment may be mediated by coping skills. For example, individuals for whom race and ethnicity are more significant spend more time thinking about race, ethnicity, and/or discrimination and develop more varied and sophisticated coping skills that are more likely to lead to favorable outcomes, and (4) the youth's *sense of meaning in their lives* mediated the relation between ethnic identity and adjustment. So, combining meaning making, cognitive appraisal, and coping, in addition to a positive identification with one's racial and ethnic identity, promotes resiliency against experiences of racism and discrimination.[50] Research has demonstrated that Mexican-American adolescents who were faced with high levels of discrimination were able to maintain high levels of self-esteem if they had high levels of *ethnic affirmation*, whereas those adolescents with low levels of ethnic affirmation seemed to suffer.[51] In turn, African American youth with a positive connection to their ethnic group seemed to be protected against poor academic achievement and problem behaviors when faced with discrimination, whereas those who did not have this connection were not.[52]

Ethnic-racial socialization refers to the process by which caregivers convey implicit and explicit messages about the significance and meaning of race and ethnicity, teach children about what it means to be a member of a racial and/or ethnic minority group, and help youth learn to cope with discrimination.[53] Primary caregivers of ethnic minority youth differ in the extent to which they engage in ethnic-racial socialization, but several studies suggest that ethnic-racial socialization is fairly common across ethnic minority families. Some of the messages caregivers transmit to their children include (1) *cultural socialization*: teaching children about their racial–ethnic heritage and history and promoting cultural, racial, and ethnic pride; (2) *preparation for bias*: highlighting the existence of inequalities between groups and preparing youth to cope with discrimination; (3) *egalitarianism:* emphasizing individual character traits such as hard work over racial or ethnic group membership; (4) *self-worth messages*: promoting feelings of individual worth within the broader context of the child's race and ethnicity; (5) *negative messages*: emphasizing negative characteristics associated with being a racial–ethnic minority; (6) *silence about race and ethnicity:* failing to mention issues pertaining to race or ethnicity; and (7) *promotion of mistrust*: conveying distrust in interracial communications. Studies across diverse groups of ethnic minority youth link ethnic-racial socialization with a broad range of positive outcomes, including academic performance, ethnic and racial identity, socioemotional adjustment, racial ideology, ethnic affirmation, and positive self-concept. However, some ethnic-racial socialization messages can also have negative outcomes[54]; for example, *preparation for bias messages*, in isolation, may contribute to low self-esteem in youth by instilling in them a sense of lack of control over their environment and leading them to disengage from academic and other pursuits. In contrast, patterns of racial socialization emphasizing both *cultural socialization* and *preparation for bias* buffered the impact that racial discrimination had on African American adolescents' perceived stress and problem behavior this may also extend to immigrant youth, underscoring how various dimensions of ethnic-racial socialization coalesce to convey meta-messages regarding the significance and meaning of race and ethnicity to youth.[46] It is safe to assume that the same patterns of cultural and racial socialization would have similar effects on immigrant children, especially if their phenotype is different from that of the members of the dominant group of the majority host culture.

Cultural orientation refers to the youth's orientations toward mainstream culture and/or to their ethnic culture and has often been explained by endorsement of particular cultural values. Research on youth who have a strong orientation toward their ethnic culture describe positive developmental outcomes such as good self-esteem, better academic engagement, positive racial self-image and psychological well-being, as well as less risk for substance abuse, depression, and externalizing behaviors. Another similar concept that has been studied in relation to immigrant and minority youth and families has been that of *familism*, which encompasses youth's sense of family identification, solidarity, cohesion, and duty, as well as support received from the family. Various aspects of *familism* have been positively associated with psychological adjustment, and its opposite, *acculturative-family-distancing*, has been associated to deviant behaviors[46] that suggest that these 3 key factors—*racial and ethnic identity*, *ethnic-racial socialization*, and *cultural orientation*—operate as protective factors against discrimination and promote youth adjustment, and they reciprocally influence one another, while simultaneously influencing and being shaped by self-concept, attributions, cognitive appraisals, and coping. *The integrative approach* about how these concepts interact with one another is explained as follows: (1) all 3 constructs are found to contribute to ethnic minority youth's perceptions of their competence and adequacy and to bolster their self-concept. (2) Each of the protective factors may play a role in the cognitive appraisal process, including how youth attend to, understand, and make sense of the world. Ethnic-racial socialization processes prepare youth to perceive the world in a certain way, whereas ethnic and racial identity and cultural orientation may inform the salience and significance of discrimination in a given context, influence attributions of personal instances of discrimination, and provide youth with a sense of meaning. (3) *Coping* seems to be a critical intermediary process in the promotion of youth outcomes. Ethnic and racial identity and ethnic-racial socialization may facilitate the development of specific adaptive coping skills that help youth to negotiate ethnic and racial discrimination. Similarly, cultural orientation and values such as *familism* may provide the support necessary to help youth to cope. In addition, positive messages about the significance and meaning of being a member of a racial or ethnic minority group and positive feelings about one's group allow youth to feel competent across multiple domains and may inform how youth experience and understand the world. (4) Youth who are more aware of discrimination due to their identity, socialization, or cultural orientation may understand a racial or ethnic affront as part of the way the world operates, rather than as a personal derogation. Being able to make sense of their surroundings informs youth how to cope with their environment. Thus, youth who feel confident, capable, and competent develop more adaptive coping strategies than do those youth who feel insecure and perceive the world as threatening. In essence, it is likely that the protective factors operate in a cyclical, rather than a linear, manner, such that they mutually influence one another across development.[50]

RECOMMENDATIONS FOR TREATING PATIENTS OF A DIFFERENT RACIAL–ETHNIC GROUP

1) Addressing the topic of race with patients is usually situation specific. Sometimes the most prudent approach is to "put the topic on the table" should it be relevant for the future. Other times, therapists and patients may find themselves involved in important conversations about the possible influence of race in the therapeutic process, yet with others the topic of race may develop slowly over time. The variables affecting how these conversations may develop include the level of the patient's trust in the therapist, the patient's understanding of his or her own racial–ethnic identity, and the overall importance that racial–ethnic issues have for a given

individual. One significant benefit of engaging in conversations about race and ethnicity with patients is that it reduces the likelihood of stereotyping and the assumption that patients possess certain group characteristics.

2) The racial–ethnic background of clients may not be obvious, especially when it involves biracial or multiracial patients or patients whose racial–ethnic identity is not obvious from physical characteristics. So it is important to suspend preconceptions about patients' race–ethnicity and that of their family members and pace the timing and sensitivity of the conversations over the course of a therapeutic relationship. Similarly, patients who have a partner or other family member from another racial or ethnic group, such as in the case of adopted family members, may appreciate efforts on the part of the therapist not to make quick assumptions about the person in question's race because using inaccurate terminology may be offensive to the patient.

3) Recognize that patients may be quite different from other patients in their racial–ethnic group.

4) Always consider how ethnic–racial differences between therapist and patient may affect the psychotherapy process, and in addition to having conversations about the patient's ethnic–racial identity, it is important to acknowledge the ethnic-racial identity of the therapist. Because these differences may affect the psychotherapy process, including differences in attitudes and expectations toward mental health services and conceptions of the self in relation to family and community, communication and interaction styles, differences in conceptualization of mental health and mental illness, and differences in the styles of verbal and nonverbal communication.

5) Acknowledging that power, privilege, and racism can affect the therapeutic process because minority patients may have experienced them more directly on a personal level and failing to acknowledge these societal issues in the context of psychotherapy could make the patient reexperience past painful personal experiences that may alienate minority patients.

6) When in doubt about the importance of race and ethnicity, err on the side of discussion. These conversations about race and ethnicity can be uncomfortable due to anxiety about offending or alienating the other person or being judged for "saying the wrong thing." In the event that the patient seems uncomfortable when a therapist raises the topic of race and ethnicity, this can be approached in the same manner as when there has been an empathic break or a disruption in the therapeutic alliance. Nevertheless, broaching issues of race and ethnicity, even if the therapist is not sure of exactly what to say, is better than ignoring the topic.[55,56]

CONCLUSIONS AND FUTURE DIRECTIONS

The United States was once a country with a large white majority population and a small black minority with impenetrable color lines, but over the past 4 decades immigration has increased the racial and ethnic diversity in the United States. Along with increased immigration are increases in the rates of ethnic/racial intermarriage, which is transforming the American landscape into one with a growing multiracial population. These trends indicate that (1) the multiracial population seems likely to continue to grow in the foreseeable future because of increasing intermarriage. (2) Multiracial identification is not uncommon among the members of new immigrant groups such as Asians and Latinos, particularly for those younger than 18 years. (3) Multiracial identification remains relatively uncommon among blacks compared with Asians and Latinos. (4) These patterns suggest that multiracial reporting is more likely in areas with greater levels of racial–ethnic diversity. (5) The increases in intermarriage and the growth of the multiracial population reflect a blending of races and the fading of color lines and perhaps a reduction in social distance and racial prejudice; these patterns seem to offer an optimistic portrait of weakening racial boundaries. (6) Yet, the continuing black-nonblack divide with ongoing racism, discrimination, ignorance, marginalization, and decreased educational and socioeconomic opportunities could be a disastrous outcome for many African Americans.[4,5] It is our responsibility as child psychiatrists and therapists to learn more about issues of race and ethnicity and about the important sociopolitical events that have occurred in American history, as well as about issues such as acculturation and identity development.

DISCLOSURE

E. M. Rothe receives book royalties from Oxford University Press. A. S. Lacay has nothing to disclose.

REFERENCES

1. Camarota S. A record-Setting decade of immigration: 2000-2010 Center for immigration studies. 2011. Available at: http://cis.org/2000-2010-record-setting-decade-immigration. Accessed Dec. 15, 2018.
2. Homeland Scurity news Wire U.S. Immigrant population at record 40 million in 2010. Monday 2021. Available at: http://www.homelandsecuritynewswire.com/us-immigrant-population-record-40-million-2010.
3. US Census. Population reports. 2014. Available at: https://www.census.gov/.
4. Rothe EM, Pumariega AJ. Immigration, cultural identity and mental health: psychosocial Implications of the Reshaping of America. Oxford University Press; 2020.
5. Lee J, Bean FD. America's changing color lines: immigration, Race/Ethnicity, and Multiracial Identification. Annu Rev Sociol 2004;30:221–42.
6. Fredrickson GM. The Arrogance of race: historical perspectives on slavery, racism, and social inequality. Middletown, CT: Wesleyan Univ. Press; 1988.
7. Schwartz SJ, Montgomery MJ, Briones E. The role of identity and acculturation among immigrant people: theoretical propositions, empirical questions, and applied recommendations. Hum Dev 2005;304:1–30.
8. Stein J, Urdang L, editors. Random House dictionary of the English language: the unabridged edition. New York: Random House; 1966.
9. Rothe EM, Tzuang D, Pumariega AJ. Acculturation, development and adaptation. Child Adolesc Psychiatr Clin N Am 2010;19(No. 4):681–96.
10. Harris DR, Sim JJ. Who is multiracial? Assessing the complexity of lived race. Am Sociol Rev 2002;67(4):614–27.
11. Gordon M. Assimilation in American life. New York: Oxford Univ. Press; 1964.
12. Portes A, Zhou M. The new second generation: segmented assimilation and its variants. Ann Am Acad Pol Soc Sci 1993;530:74–96.
13. Portes A, Rumbaut RG. Legacies: the story of the immigrant second generation. Berkeley: Univ. Calif. Press; 2001.
14. Anderson M, Lopez MH, Rohal M. A rising share of the U.S. Black population is foreign born: 9% are immigrants and while most are from the Caribbean, Africans drive recent growth. Pew Research Center; 2015. Available at: https://www.pewresearch.org/fact-tank/2018/01/24/key-facts-about-black-immigrants-in-the-u-s/. Accessed September 12, 2019.

15. Thomas KJA. A demographic profile of black Caribbean immigrants in the United States. Migration Policy Institute; 2012. Available at: https://www.migrationpolicy. org/research/CBI-demographic-profile-black-caribbean-immigrants. Accessed September 12, 2019.

16. Manuel R, Taylor RJ, Jackson JS. Race and ethnic group differences in socio-economic status: black Caribbeans, African Americans and non-Hispanic whites in the United States Western. J Black Stud 2012;36:228–39.

17. Thornton M, Taylor RJ, Chatters LM. African Americans and black Caribbean mutual feelings of closeness: findings from a national Probability Survey. J Black Stud 2013;44(8):798–828.

18. A singular population: Indian-Americans in America. Chazen Global Insights. Available at: https://www8.gsb.columbia.edu/articles/chazen-global-insights/ singular-population-indian-immigrants-america.

19. Chandres KV, Chandres SV, DeLambo DA. Counseling Asian American Indians from India: Implication for training multicultural counselors ideas in research you can Use. Vistas. 2013. Available at: https://www.counseling.org/knowledge-center/vistas/by-subject2/vistas-multicultural-issues/docs/default-source/vistas/ counseling-asian-american-indians-from-india—implications-for-training-multicultural-counselors.

20. Asian American/Pacific islander communities and mental health. Mental health in America. 2021. Available at: https://www.mhanational.org/issues/asian-americanpacific-islander-communities-and-mental-health.

21. Javier JR, Supan J, Lansang A, et al. Preventing Filipino mental health Disparities: Perspectives from adolescents, caregivers, providers, and advocates. Asian Am Psychol 2014;5(4):316–24.

22. Alba RD. Ethnic identity: the Transformation of white America. New Haven, CT: Yale Univ. Press; 1990.

23. Waters MC. Ethnic Options: Choosing identities in America. Berkeley: Univ. Calif. Press; 1990.

24. Lee J, Bean FD. Beyond black and white: remaking race in America. Contexts 2003;2(3):26–33.

25. Perlmann J. Reflecting the changing face of America: multiracials, racial classification, and American intermarriage. In: Sollars W, editor. Interracialism:.Black-White intermarriage in American history, Literature, and law. New York: Oxford Univ. Press; 2000. p. 506–33.

26. Davis FJ. Who is black? One nation's definition. University Park: Penn. State Univ. Press; 1991.

27. Spencer JM. The new colored people: the mixed-race Movement in America. New York: New York Univ. Press; 1997.

28. Pumariega AJ, Joshi S. Culture and development in children and youth. Child Adolesc Psychiatr Clin N Am 2010;19(No.4):661–80.

29. Vonk ME. Cultural competence for transracial adoptive parents. Soc Work 2001; 46(3):246–55.

30. Portes A, Schlauffer R. Language and the second generation: bilingualism yesterday and today. In: Portes A, editor. The new second generation. New York: Russel-Sage; 1996. p. 28.

31. Portes A, Rumbaut RG. Immigrant America: a portrait. 2nd edition. Berkeley (CA): University of California Press; 1997.

32. Waters MC, Kasinitz P, Asad LA. Immigrants and African Americans. Annu Rev Sociol 2014;40:369–90.

33. Stepick A, Stepick CD. Power and identity: Miami Cubans. In: Suárez Orozco MM, Páez M, editors. Latinos: Remaking America. Cambridge, MA: Harvard University Press; 2002. p. 75–92.

34. U.S. Census Bureau. 2019. Available at: https://www.census.gov/.

35. Seaton EK, Caldwell CH, Sellers RM, et al. The prevalence of perceived discrimination among African American and Caribbean Black youth. Dev Psychol 2008; 44:1288–97.

36. Perez D, Fortuna L, Alegria M. Prevalence and correlates of everyday discrimination among U.S. Latinos. J Community Psychol 2008;36:421–33.

37. Hersch J. Profiling the new immigrant worker: the effects of skin color and height. J Labor Econ 2008;26(2):345–86.

38. Hersh J. The persistence of skin color discrimination for immigrants. Soc Sci Res 2011;40:1337–49.

39. Adams EA, Kurz-Costes BE, Hoffman AJ. Skin tone bias among African Americans: Antecedents and consequences across the life span. Dev Rev 2016;40: 93–116.

40. Hill M. Skin color and the perception of attractiveness among African Americans: does gender make a difference? Soc Psychol Q 2002;65:77–91.

41. Marrow HB. New immigrant destinations and the American colour line. Ethn Racial Stud 2009;32(6):1037–57.

42. Bonilla-Silva E. We are all Americans! : the Latin Americanization of racial stratification in the USA. Race Soc 2002;5:3–16.

43. Jones CP. Levels of racism: a theoretic framework and a gardener's tale. Am J Public Health 2000;90:1212–5.

44. Williams DR, Yu Y, Jackson JS, et al. Racial differences in physical and mental health socio-economic status, stress and discrimination. J Health Psychol 1997;2:335–51.

45. Molina KM, Drexler J. Discrimination, internalized racism, and depression: a comparative study of African American and Afro-Caribbean adults in the U.S. Group Processes & Intergroup Relations 2016;19(4):439–61.

46. Thornton MC, Taylor RJ, Chatters LM. African American and black Caribbean mutual feelings of closeness: findings from a national Probability Survey. J Black Stud 2013;44:798–828.

47. Cobb CL, Meca A, Branscome N, et al. Perceived discrimination and well-being among unauthorized Hispanic immigrants: the Moderating role of ethnic/racial group identity centrality. Cultural diversity and ethnic minority Psychology. 2018. Available at: https://www.researchgate.net/publication/326426415. Accessed June 1st 2019.

48. Cross WE, Parham TA, Helms JE. Nigrescence revisited: Theory and research. In: Jones RL, editor. African American identity development: Theory, research, and intervention. Hampton, (VA): Cobb and Henry; 1998.

49. Perkins K, Wiley S, Deaux K. Through which looking Glass? Distinct sources of Public regard and self-esteem among first- and second-generation immigrants of color. Cultur Divers Ethnic Minor Psychol 2014;20(No. 2):213–9.

50. Neblett EW, White RL, Ford KR, Philip CL, et al. Patterns of racial socialization and psychological adjustment: can parental communications about race reduce the impact of racial discrimination? J Res Adolescence 2008;18:477–515.

51. Romero AJ, Roberts RE. The impact of multiple dimensions of ethnic identity on discrimination and adolescents' self-esteem. J Appl Soc Psychol 2003;33: 2288–305.

52. Wong CA, Eccles JS, Sameroff A. The influence of ethnic discrimination and ethnic identification on African American adolescents' school and socioemotional adjustment. J Pers 2003;71:1197–232.
53. Hughes D, Rodriguez J, Smith EP, et al. Parents' ethnic-racial socialization practices: a review of research and directions for future study. Dev Psychol 2006;42: 747–70.
54. Hughes D, Witherspoon D, Rivas-Drake D, West-Bey N. Received ethnic-racial socialization messages and youth's academic and behavioral outcomes: Examining the mediating role of ethnic identity and self-esteem. Cultur Divers Ethnic Minor Psychol 2009;15:112–24.
55. Cardemil EV, Battle CL. Guess Who's coming to therapy? Getting Comfortable with conversations about race and ethnicity in psychotherapy. professional Psychology: research and practice. Copyright 2003 by Am Psychol Assoc Inc. 2003; 34(No. 3):278–86.
56. Sue DW, Sue D. Counseling the culturally diverse: Theory and practice. 4th ed. New York: Wiley; 2003.

Printed and bound by CPI Group (UK) Ltd, Croydon, CR0 4YY

03/10/2024

01040467-0015